On the Measurement
of Human Fertility

A Population Council Book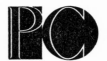

On the Measurement of Human Fertility

*Selected Writings
of Louis Henry*

TRANSLATED AND EDITED BY

Mindel C. Sheps
*Department of Biostatistics
University of North Carolina*

Evelyne Lapierre-Adamcyk
The Population Council

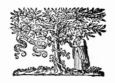

Elsevier Publishing Company
AMSTERDAM • LONDON • NEW YORK
1972

Elsevier Publishing Company
335 Jan van Galenstraat
P.O. Box 211, Amsterdam, The Netherlands

American Elsevier Publishing Company, Inc.
52 Vanderbilt Avenue
New York, New York 10017

Library of Congress Catalog Card Number: 72-76712
ISBN 0-444-41029-5

Printed in the United States of America

Preface

INVESTIGATION OF the determinants of human natality levels is a major component of the study of population growth and change. While social, economic, and psychological factors are the principal sources of variation in natality, they can operate only within the confines and context of the physiological determinants of reproduction. Their influence is exerted through modifying one or more physiological factors.

It is therefore important to investigate how and to what extent natural and induced variation in physiological functions affects human reproduction. Important avenues for such investigations are analysis of data from populations reproducing "naturally" (i.e., without taking actions deliberately intended to limit births) and formulation of models that clarify the effects of the physiological functions in question.

The first sustained and extensive investigation of such models was undertaken by Professor Louis Henry, of the University of Paris. His work, published as a series of papers, appeared over the course of 15 years. The models are intended primarily to investigate problems arising in the analysis of the reproductive performance of married women. Stimulated by his demographic analyses of old family and parish records, Professor Henry in effect formulated a series of questions, the answers to which were far from obvious. Some of these questions are:

1) What is the variation in "natural fertility" of humans, i.e., the variation in the reproductive patterns of married couples who do not deliberately limit their reproduction by resorting to contraception or induced abortion?

2) What is the role of the principal biological determinants of reproduction in this variation?

3) Given a collection of family histories, with data on the date of marriage, the age of the couple at marriage, and the number of births and the date of each successive birth, how can one establish the most informative methods of analyzing the data? What inferences can be made about the natural fecundity of the couples, about variation with age in the biological determinants, about differences between groups,

or about the time when a defined population began to turn to contraception?

To pursue such questions, Professor Henry formulated mathematical models for the process of *family building,* i.e., for the process
that results in a sequence of births to a married woman, spaced apart
by intervals of measurable length. These models and the conclusions
drawn from them are presented in his papers translated here.

The results are fascinating and important. Our understanding of
the sources of variation in observed data and of possible pitfalls in
analysis has been considerably advanced by Professor Henry's pioneer-
ing efforts. Previously, limited aspects of the problems he investigated
had been considered by Corrado Gini in Italy and Raymond Pearl
in the United States. Subsequently, the field of family building models
has been explored not only by French investigators but by a number
of workers writing in English, only some of whom had benefited from
Professor Henry's work. Some of his results have been rediscovered,
but many are still not known to the majority of English-speaking investigators.

The translations were first undertaken informally, for the benefit
of a small group of colleagues and students. Having learned a great
deal in the process, we felt that these papers should be made more
accessible to those who understand English better than they do French.
Happily, the Population Council willingly cooperated by making it
possible for Evelyne Lapierre-Adamcyk to serve as coeditor and by
including the translation in its publication schedule.

The principal objective of the translation is to present Professor
Henry's thoughts accurately. Our efforts were expanded mainly in a
careful checking for such accuracy. We were greatly aided by his
careful perusal of two drafts of the translations and by his patient
explanations and clarifications in reply to the numerous questions
we addressed to him. As a result, author's corrections, editors' corrections, and occasional footnotes have been added. The editors' addi-
tions and corrections in the text are enclosed in square brackets; the
author's are identified "—L.H." and enclosed in square brackets.

We acknowledge with thanks those who assisted in the translations.
First drafts were contributed by Emily Greenspan, by Jean Pierre
Biné, and by William Haenszel of the National Cancer Institute who
arranged for translations of the papers published in 1957 and 1961
(Chapters Two and Three). Professor Nathan Keyfitz gave us helpful
comments on a preliminary English version. Jane A. Menken and C.
Suchindran read the whole manuscript carefully and made many im-

portant suggestions. During the first part of the work, which was carried out at Columbia University, Annette P. Radick assumed major supervisory responsibility. She rendered invaluable service in checking the translations and the mathematics, and was generally responsible for managing the many essential details related to the preparation and correction of successive drafts.

For the laborious effort of repeated typing of a difficult manuscript, we thank Marlene Brodas and Doris Johnson of Columbia University and Liliane Cusson in Montreal.

For financial support, we owe thanks to a Ford Foundation grant to the International Institute for the Study of Human Reproduction at Columbia University, to the Department of Biostatistics at the University of North Carolina, and to the Population Council.

Any errors or other shortcomings that may remain in this book are completely our responsibility. We hope that, despite such shortcomings, the book will serve a useful purpose by introducing Louis Henry's work to the wider audience it so clearly deserves.

Chapel Hill, N.C.   M.C.S.
New York, N.Y.   E.L-A.

January 1972

List of Tables

List of Figures

Contents

On the Measurement
of Human Fertility

CHAPTER ONE

Theoretical Basis
of Measures of Natural Fertility*

EDITORS' SUMMARY

This paper (published in 1953) presents a family building model that does not have explicit provisions for pregnancy wastage. Fecundability (here defined as the probability of a conception leading to a live birth) and the duration of the nonsusceptible period are allowed to vary between couples but are assumed to be constant for each couple, before the onset of definitive sterility. The model provides for the incidence of sterility to increase with age. On these assumptions, results are derived for the expected fertility rate and the expected cumulative fertility at a duration x *of marriage. Methods of estimating the relevant parameters from empirical data on family building are discussed, as well as biases that may arise in different kinds of data.*

Originally printed in French as "Fondements théoriques des mesures de la fécondité naturelle." Revue de l'Institut International de Statistique 21, no. 3 (1953): 135–151.

CONTENTS

INTRODUCTION

One of the most interesting and difficult problems in demography is that of estimating natural fertility, i.e. the fertility of a human population that makes no deliberate effort to limit births. Natural fertility, which depends essentially on biological factors, is primarily a biological phenomenon, and a "natural" phenomenon has a particular attraction. It shares in the prestige of the natural sciences, overshadowing that of the social sciences which are still in their infancy. In addition, efforts to appraise the effectiveness of contraceptive practice lead to comparisons between actual fertility and the hypothetical fertility that a given population would have if it did not use any form of birth control.

The difficulties encountered in the study of natural fertility result from its very definition. Natural fertility is, for easily observable populations, hypothetical. No doubt one can find populations living under conditions of quasi-natural fertility; but, for the most part, little is known about them. For European populations, before the spread of contraceptive practice, only scanty data are available.

Thus, it is not surprising that indirect approaches are made to circumvent the difficulty. But in following indirect routes we risk losing sight of the goal: An investigation of the theoretical basis of measures of natural fertility is indispensable.

SUMMARY OF NOTATION

g	Duration of nonsusceptibility associated with pregnancy (i.e. gestation plus postpartum nonsusceptible period).
g_0	Duration of pregnancy.
$h(g)$	Probability density function (p.d.f.) of g.
$\bar{g}$	Mean of g.
$\bar{g}_h$	Harmonic mean of g.
p	Fecundability in the discrete case, i.e. probability of conceiving per menstrual cycle.
$f(p)$	P.d.f. of p.
$\bar{p}$	Mean fecundability in the discrete case.
c	Coefficient of variation of p.
i	Mean interval between births in a homogeneous group.
$\bar{\imath}$	Mean interval between births in a heterogeneous group of fecund women.
$\bar{\imath}'$	Mean interval between births in a heterogeneous group of women in the presence of sterility.
ϕ	Fecundability in the continuous case, i.e. instantaneous risk of conceiving.
$f(\phi)$	P.d.f. of ϕ.
$\bar{\phi}$	Mean fecundability in the continuous case.
$\bar{\phi}_h$	Harmonic mean of ϕ.
ϕ'	Asymptotic fertility rate (i.e. $\phi' = 1/i$), homogeneous case for fecund women.
$\bar{\phi}'$	Corresponding fertility rate in a heterogeneous group.
$k(\phi')$	P.d.f. of ϕ'.
$B(x)$	Instantaneous fertility rate at time x.
x	Duration of marriage.
x_0	Age at marriage (real or translated).
$u(x_0, x)$	Mean duration of fecund years in a marriage between x_0 and x.
u_{x_0}	Mean number of fecund years per completed marriage, where the marriage occurs at x_0.
$F(x_0 + x)$	Proportion of married women who are fecund at age $x_0 + x$.
$F'(x)$	Proportion of married women still fecund x years after the preceding birth.

dS	Instantaneous risk of becoming sterile.
$E(x)$	Cumulative fertility at time x, i.e. expected number of children born in x years of marriage.
E_0	Intercept for the approximation:
	$$E(x) \approx E_0 + x\phi'.$$
E_{x_0}	Completed fertility of women married at x_0.

We will start with certain assumptions regarding the biological basis of fertility. These assumptions are not completely arbitrary; observed results are used to construct a mathematical model that is as close to reality as possible and yet simple enough to be easily manageable.

FUNDAMENTAL ASSUMPTIONS

It has long since been ascertained that in large families of a fixed size, the interval between successive births is more or less independent of birth order, except perhaps for the last few births. Now, a priori, the interval between births depends on the duration of pregnancy (independent of order), on the duration of the nonsusceptible period that follows confinement, and on the natural fecundity of the couple. If the mean interval between successive births does not vary, it is natural to think that these various factors also do not vary for a given couple as long as they are not sterile.

We were led, therefore, to characterize each fecund couple (couple able to produce living children, at the time or later):

1. by the duration, g, of the nonsusceptible period associated with pregnancy; g is the time that elapses between a conception and the first ovulation after delivery.

2. by fecundability or the probability of conception per unit time outside of the previously mentioned nonsusceptible periods.

Since conception is possible only at the time of ovulation, one ought, rigorously, to treat fecundability as discrete and define it as the probability of conceiving per menstrual cycle. In this case we designate it by p. But since it is often more convenient to treat time as continuous, we also introduce the probability ϕdx of conceiving during the infinitely small time interval dx. The term fecundability is also used for ϕ.

The quantity g is the sum of two terms: the duration of pregnancy, g_0, and the duration, $g-g_0$, of the period of nonsusceptibility following delivery. The latter varies appreciably between women, because, while it is very short in the absence of breast-feeding, it can be very long in the case of prolonged lactation. Moreover, fecundability certainly varies between women, whether because of the physiological characteristics of the couple or of the frequency of their sexual relations. To take these variations into account, we introduce two distributions: $h(g)$, the probability density function (p.d.f.) of the duration of nonsusceptibility, and $f(\phi)$, the p.d.f. of fecundability, or $f(p)$ in the discrete case.

Before going on, let us examine the foregoing. To characterize each couple by a pair (ϕ,g), is to assume that these quantities are invariant in time as long as the couple is not definitely sterile. It is certain that, in reality, ϕ and g vary over time. For g, this is obvious. Illness of the mother or death of the child may interrupt lactation; furthermore, if one considers conceptions, the duration of pregnancy also varies.[1]

It is more difficult to affirm, a priori, that ϕ varies. Doubtless our sense of continuity makes us think that women do not become completely sterile suddenly, without a preceding progressive decline in fecundability. But this feeling for continuity, though undeniable, does not constitute an argument. One could object to the assumption of a constant ϕ on the grounds of the existence of nonsusceptible periods outside of those associated with pregnancy, e.g. those due to separation or illness. But to the extent that these separations and illnesses are distributed uniformly in time, they intervene by modifying the probability of conception; they do not affect its assumed invariance.

On the other hand, we must admit that the distribution of these separations and illnesses is certainly not uniform. Long established marriages accept temporary separations more easily

---

[1] In the case of spontaneous abortion, pregnancy is shorter. For convenience, we often operate as if there were a fixed time between conception and birth and pass from one to the other at our choice. We are not unaware, however, that the existence of spontaneous abortions and stillbirths complicates matters. But these are secondary difficulties which it appears unnecessary to expound here.

than do young married couples; also, the frequency of illness increases with age and therefore with duration of marriage. Thus, separations and illnesses tend to lower ϕ with increasing duration of marriage.

The relatively small variation in observed mean intervals between successive births shows, however, that variations in ϕ and g depend little on the duration of marriage, age or parity. With respect to g, this suggests that if this function varies for a given couple, the variation is independent of the duration of marriage. On the average, g will be the same at any point in a marriage. We shall see that under these conditions, the results are the same as if we assume a constant g for each couple.

REPRODUCTIVE HISTORY
OF A GROUP OF COUPLES

We begin by considering the reproductive history of a group of couples with the same characteristics (ϕ,g) in the absence of permanent sterility and of dissolution of the marriage by separation, divorce or death.

It is natural to take marriage as the time origin, under the assumption of no premarital sexual relations and, hence, no premarital conceptions. But, on this assumption, the period from marriage to the first live birth (if, as we are doing, one considers live births only) differs from subsequent intervals because g_0, the duration of pregnancy, rather than g, intervenes in this first interval. One could, obviously, retain this difference, but only at the cost of complicating the notation. It is simpler to change the origin, placing it at $g-g_0$ before marriage.

Let us designate the elapsed time from this translated origin by x. For $x<g$, all couples are childless; for $x>g$, the expected number of couples without births, taking the initial sample size as unity, is equal to $e^{-\phi(x-g)}$ and the number of first births in the interval $(x,x+dx)$ is $\phi e^{-\phi(x-g)}dx$.

For $x<2g$, there are no second order births; it can easily be shown that, for $x\geqslant2g$, the expected number in the interval $(x,x+dx)$ is equal to $\phi^2(x-2g)e^{-\phi(x-2g)}dx$.

It is then easy to show by recursion that, for $x\geqslant ng$, the expected number of births of order n in the interval $(x,x+dx)$ is equal to[2]

$$\phi^n \frac{(x-ng)^{n-1}}{(n-1)!} e^{-\phi(x-ng)} dx. \tag{1}$$

The expected number of births $B(x)dx$ in the interval $(x,x+dx)$, regardless of order, is equal to the sum of (1) for values of n from 1 to m such that $mg \leqslant x$. $B(x)$ is given by:

$$B(x) = \int_g^\infty B(x-t)\phi e^{-\phi(t-g)} dt \tag{2}$$

which is of the same form as equations studied by Lotka. Its solution is of the form $\sum_s Q_s e^{r_s x}$. The Q_s are coefficients and the r_s are roots of the equation

$$1 = \int_g^\infty \phi e^{-rt-\phi(t-g)} dt. \tag{3}$$

The real root is zero and the real component of the imaginary roots is negative. Consequently, $B(x)$ is the sum of a constant and of damped periodic functions. With increasing duration of marriage, this sum approaches the constant part of $B(x)$, which we designate by ϕ' (asymptotic fertility rate). This is equal to $1/i$, where i is the mean interval between births. Now.

$$i = \int_g^\infty \phi x e^{-\phi(x-g)} dx = g + \int_g^\infty \phi(x-g)e^{-\phi(x-g)} dx \tag{4}$$

whence $i = g + \dfrac{1}{\phi}$. Hence

$$\phi' = \frac{1}{g+1/\phi} = \frac{\phi}{1+g\phi}. \tag{5}$$

Often in demography, rates are only intermediate results in the attempt to derive the mean number of events per capita over a long period: here, the mean number of births per marriage.

---

[2] If one had considered couples with fecundability ϕ and $g_0, \ldots g_{n-1}$ for the duration of nonsusceptability corresponding to each successive birth order, one would have obtained for the number of births of order n in the interval $(x,x+dx)$:

$$\phi^n \frac{(x-g_0-g_1-\cdots-g_{n-1})^{n-1}}{(n-1)!} e^{-\phi(x-g_0-g_1-\cdots-g_{n-1})} dx,$$

for $x \geqslant g_0+g_1+\cdots+g_{n-1}$, given that g_k is not dependent upon the duration of marriage. For a set of couples in which $g_0+g_1+\cdots+g_{n-1}=ng$, we again arrive at the earlier result. There is no need, therefore, to introduce variations of g independent of marital duration.

Hence, we are led to study cumulative fertility as a function of time, that is, the expected number of children born in x years of marriage. Let us designate it by $E(x)$. We have:

$$E(x) = \int_0^x B(\zeta)d\zeta = \phi' x + \sum_s \int_0^x Q_s e^{rs\zeta} d\zeta. \tag{6}$$

$E(x)$ is the sum of a linear function of x and of damped periodic functions. After a number of oscillations, that is, after a given duration of marriage, $E(x)$ approaches $\phi'x+E_o$, where E_o depends on ϕ and g. Given ϕ and g, $E(x)$ can be calculated from appropriate tables, e.g. χ^2 tables [since Eq. (1) is equivalent to a χ^2 (chi square) distribution with $2n$ degrees of freedom]. From this, one deduces E_o. But it is not necessary to consider all pairs (ϕ,g). Let us assume two values, g and λg. The maximum value of n in time x given g is the same as the maximum value in time λx given λg. If ϕ is the fecundability associated with g, let us consider the pair $(\phi/\lambda,\lambda g)$. We then have:

$$E(x|\phi,g) = \sum_1^n \int_{ng}^x \frac{\phi^n(\xi-ng)^{n-1}}{(n-1)!} e^{-\phi(\xi-ng)} d\xi \tag{7}$$

$$E(\lambda x|\phi/\lambda, \lambda g) = \sum_1^n \int_{\lambda ng}^{\lambda x} \left(\frac{\phi}{\lambda}\right)^n \frac{(\zeta-\lambda ng)^{n-1}}{(n-1)!} e^{-(\phi/\lambda)(\zeta-\lambda ng)} d\zeta. \tag{8}$$

Let $\zeta = \lambda\xi$; it follows that $E(\lambda x,/\phi/\lambda,\lambda g) = E(x,|\phi,g)$. The two

terms in x are equal to $\dfrac{\phi}{1+g\phi} x$ for the pair (ϕ,g), and to

$$\frac{\phi}{\lambda(1+g\phi)} \lambda x$$

for the pair $(\phi/\lambda,\lambda g)$. They are therefore equal and we have finally, $E_o(\phi,g) = E_o(\phi/\lambda,\lambda g)$. Hence, when $g\phi$ is a constant, E_o is fixed. Values of E_o for selected $g\phi$ were calculated, and a regression fitted as:

$$E_o = -0.5 + \frac{0.115}{g\phi}. \tag{9}$$

Table 1 shows calculated and estimated values.

TABLE 1

E_0 ACCORDING TO $g\phi$

$g\phi$	0.5	1	2	3	4	5	6	∞
E_0 calculated	−0.275	−0.375	−0.445	−0.470	−0.480	−0.485	−0.490	−0.500
E_0 estimated from Eq. (9)	−0.270	[−0.385]	−0.443	−0.462	−0.471	−0.477	−0.481	−0.500

We now pass to the more realistic case of a heterogeneous group where the couples have all possible characteristics (ϕ,g). Assume that there is no correlation between ϕ and g; the group is then characterized by two probability densities, $f(\phi)$ and $h(g)$. This group, by virtue of the heterogeneity of ϕ and g, has diverse values for ϕ'; the distribution of ϕ' has a probability density $k(\phi')$.

In such a group, the expected number of births in the interval $(x, x+dx)$ is equal to the sum of the births of the homogeneous subgroups (ϕ,g) which constitute the entire group. If x is large, the expected number in the subgroup (ϕ,g) departs little from $\phi'dx$; the expected number of births for the total, therefore, is equal to $dx \int \phi'k(\phi')d\phi' = \bar{\phi}'dx$, and the cumulative fertility of the group is approximately equal to

$$x \int \phi'k(\phi')d\phi' + \int \int E_0 f(\phi)h(g)d\phi dg \qquad (10)$$

or $x\bar{\phi}'+\bar{E}_0$, where $\bar{E}_0$ is the mean of the values of E_0 corresponding to the various combinations (ϕ,g).

If we substitute Eq. (9), the approximation for E_0 referring to a sufficiently long time, into Eq. (10), the result is:

$$\bar{E}_0 = -0.500 + 0.115 \int \frac{f(\phi)d\phi}{\phi} \int \frac{h(g)dg}{g} = -0.500 + \frac{0.115}{\bar{\phi}_h \bar{g}_h}, \qquad (11)$$

where $\bar{\phi}_h$ and $\bar{g}_h$ are the harmonic means of ϕ and of g.

INTRODUCTION OF STERILITY

The proportion of sterile couples varies greatly with the woman's age. One may, not unreasonably, consider age as the only variable on which sterility depends. Let us first consider a homogeneous group (ϕ,g) and let us designate by $F(x_0+x)$ the proportion of married women still fecund at age x_0+x, where x_0 is the [translated] age at marriage. The number of births of order n occurring during the interval $(x, x+dx)$ are

$$\left(\phi^n\right)\frac{(x-ng)^{n-1}}{(n-1)!}\, e^{-\phi(x-ng)}F(x_0 + x)dx. \qquad (12)$$

The value for each birth order, and hence for their sum, is multiplied by $F(x_0+x)$. Therefore:

$$B(x) = \phi'F(x_0 + x) + \sum_s Q_s\, e^{rsx}\, F(x_0 + x) \qquad (13)$$

and

$$E(x) = \phi' \int_0^x F(x_0 + \zeta)d\zeta + \sum_s \int_0^x Q_s e^{rs\zeta}F(x_0 + \zeta)d\zeta. \qquad (14)$$

$\int_0^x F(x_0+\zeta)d\zeta$ is the mean number of years lived between the ages of x_0 and x_0+x before permanent sterility; it is, in effect, the mean duration of fecund marriage, $u(x_0,x)$, given a total duration equal to x.

In the absence of sterility, cumulative fertility presents damped oscillations around the straight line $\phi'x+E_0$. The first consequence of the intervention of sterility is to multiply the expected number of births by $F(x_0)$, the proportion of married women fecund at marriage. The progression of sterility with time causes cumulative fertility to deviate increasingly from $\phi'x+E_0$, but it seems natural that the resulting curve should continue to pass through the same origin. For the group of couples, expected cumulative fertility is therefore given by:

$$E(x) = F(x_0)\left[\phi'\frac{u(x_0, x)}{F(x_0)} + E_0\right] = \phi'u(x_0, x) + E_0F(x_0). \qquad (15)$$

In the absence of sterility, x must be sufficiently large so that $E(x) = \phi'x+E_0$. If sterility supervenes, completed fertility is limited to that achieved when all the women have become sterile. It is therefore indispensable to verify that the completed fertility E_{x_0}, is given by the above approximate formula, at least when the age at marriage, x_0, is not too close to the ages where sterility progresses rapidly.

We have attempted this verification using two ages at marriage, 25 and 35 years, with $\phi = 2.5$ and $g = 2$ [in units of one year], values which ought to be close to the mean of ϕ and g under conditions of natural fertility. We have utilized the table of $F(x)$ published in a recent work (Henry, [1], p. 99). The discrepancy between the theoretical value of ϕ' (0.417) and that obtained by the formula

$$\phi' = \frac{E_{x_0} - E_0 F(x_0)}{u_{x_0}} \tag{16}$$

is insignificant, since one finds, for $x_0 = 25$, $\phi' = 0.418$ and for $x_0 = 35$, $\phi' = 0.416$.

This verification based on completed fertility permits us to affirm that, given a sufficiently long period before all the women become sterile, the cumulative fertility for a sufficiently large x is approximated well by Eq. (15). It follows that between two marital durations, x_1 and x_2, one has:

$$E(x_2) - E(x_1) = \phi'[u(x_0, x_2) - u(x_0, x_1)]. \tag{17}$$

One can always reduce the interval (x_1, x_2) sufficiently so that $F(x_0 + x)$ is linear within the interval. It then follows that:

$$E(x_2) - E(x_1) = \phi'(x_2 - x_1)F\left(x_0 + \frac{x_1 + x_2}{2}\right). \tag{18}$$

Assume that the progression of sterility is independent of fertility ϕ'; we can then write for all values of ϕ', denoting the mean value of $E(x_2) - E(x_1)$ by $\overline{\Delta E}$:

$$\frac{\overline{\Delta E}}{x_2 - x_1} = \overline{\phi}' F\left(x_0 + \frac{x_1 + x_2}{2}\right). \tag{19}$$

This formula was obtained on the assumption that ϕ and g and, consequently, ϕ' do not vary with the age of the woman or the duration of marriage. From empirical observations, it seems that this assumption is reasonably correct only as a first approximation. It appears, according to the scanty information at our disposal, that ϕ diminishes slowly with increasing age or duration of marriage. As is the case when ϕ is invariant, births per unit time should present oscillations at first, which should then become damped. However, except for the entirely theoretical case where g is zero, it is difficult to express the expected fertility rate at duration x as a function of fecundability, which is itself a function of x, and of g. But one can always use Eq. (19): the mean fertility $\overline{\phi}'$ at duration x, now a function of x, is, by definition, the legitimate fertility at age $[x_0 + x]$ of couples fecund at this age.

MEASURES OF NATURAL FERTILITY
OF FECUND COUPLES

In Eq. (19), $\dfrac{\overline{\Delta E}}{x_2-x_1}$ is the expected natural marital fertility, or
the annual number of births per married woman, fecund or sterile, in a noncontracepting population. In practice, it may be difficult to estimate this quantity because there are few appropriate data available concerning noncontracepting populations; but in theory it is quite simple.

If ϕ' were absolutely invariant, it would then be easy to determine its value, using the annual number of births and the fact that $F(x)$ is almost equal to unity for low values of x. Even given a relatively large error in the estimate of $(1-F(x))$, the proportion of sterile couples, ϕ' would be known with adequate precision. $F(x)$ at higher ages could then be estimated using values of ϕ'.

Since the invariance of ϕ', which in any case is only an approximation, is a hypothesis to be verified, it is necessary to operate as if ϕ' varied and then proceed to determine ϕ' for diverse ages, and therefore for values of $F(x)$ not close to unity.

If one has a table of values of $F(x)$, a simple division yields an estimate of $\phi'(x)$. [In what follows, the variable x is to be understood.] This procedure is inconvenient because a direct estimate of F, difficult enough, leads only to approximations; differences in estimates of ϕ' could then be due to errors in F.

It is therefore preferable to attempt to estimate ϕ' directly. For this purpose, it is necessary to work with estimates for couples still fecund at a given age of the woman. Since this would include all couples who have births after this age, it is tempting to replace the determination of ϕ' by that of fertility between x_1 and x_2, for example, between age 25 and 30, of married women who give birth after 30. Among married women still fecund at age 30, those of low fecundity have more chance of not having more births than do those of high fecundity. Therefore, the mean fertility of married women who have children after age 30 is greater than that of married women still fecund at 30 years. Since the mean age at sterility of women who are fecund at 30 is considerably above age 30, the error of equating married women fecund at 30 to married women giving birth after age 30 is small. It seems to us that this reasoning holds up to almost 40 years of age. After age 40, the progression of sterility is rapid and women who give birth after 40 certainly have a mean fertility above that of women still fecund at 40 years. It appears prudent, therefore, not to use the above mentioned procedure[3] without precautions after the age of 40.

Knowledge of $\bar{\phi}'$ permits determination of F. One can then obtain $\bar{\phi}'$ and F up to age 40. Beyond this age the problem is more complicated; one can, however, determine the fertility at ages 40–44 of married women giving birth after the age of 45. This overestimates the fertility, at ages 40–44, of women still fecund at age 45. It can suggest changes that occur in the fertility of fecund couples when the woman is more than 40 years old. Since a precise estimate seems difficult, we must be content for the time being with approximations; because of the formula used we recapture on F what we lose on $\bar{\phi}'$. In a way, this limits the damage, although, in theory, $\bar{\phi}'$ and F do not play the same role.

The foregoing method assumes that one knows the woman's age at the birth of all her children. To date, no survey has provided this information, but it can be obtained either in studies such as Pearl [1] made twenty years ago, or by reconstructing historical families from various documents (parish registers, family records, etc.).

In a census of a population practicing little contraception (as in the English census of 1911 for women married before 1870) one can, despite the absence of information on the age of the women at their deliveries, calculate a mean value for $\bar{\phi}'$ if one has data on completed families according to parity and age at marriage. The study of parity progression ratios permits construction of a table of the function F (Henry [1]). If x_0 is the translated age at marriage (i.e. the age at $(g-g_0)$ before real marriage), and E_{x_0} the corresponding completed fertility, we have, on the assumption that $\bar{\phi}'$ is constant,

$$\bar{\phi}' = \frac{\bar{E}_{x_0} - \bar{E}_0 F(x_0)}{u_{x_0}} \text{ with } \bar{E}_0 \approx -0.500 + \frac{0.115}{\bar{\phi}_h \bar{g}_h}. \qquad (20)$$

$1/\bar{\phi}_h$ is equal to the mean interval between marriage and the first conception of a live-born child; it is of the order of one year. As for $\bar{g}_h$, it is greater than nine months and less than $\bar{g}$. Now,

---

[3] Pearl [1] utilized this procedure in a slightly different form. He determined the fertility in younger age groups of women having given birth in each age group: for example, the fertility in groups aged 20–24, 25–29, 30–34, of women married before 20 years and 35–39 years old at the time of the survey which was conducted immediately after delivery.

in a noncontracepting population, in which breast-feeding lasts fairly long, $\bar{g}$ ought to be of the order of 1.50–1.75 years; $\bar{g}_h$ should therefore be about 1.25–1.50 years. $\bar{E}_0$ is then probably between −0.400 and −0.425. As for x_0, it is equal to the actual age at marriage minus $\bar{g}-g_0$, i.e. about one year. If only young marital ages are considered, E_{x_0} is large and the relative error due to imprecision of $\bar{g}$ and E_0 is small.

It is possible to simplify further and to suppress the passage to the translated age. In the absence of sterility one would have $E_{x_0} \approx x\phi'-0.4$. It seems that ϕ' is itself little different from 0.4 for many populations, hence $E_{x_0} \approx (x-1)\phi'$. But since $(g-g_0)$ is close to one year, $x-1$ represents the actual duration of marriage. After introducing sterility as a factor, we write, with x_r the actual age at marriage, $\phi' = \bar{E}_{x_r}/u_{x_r}$.

Actually, ϕ' is not constant; it probably decreases with age, and, therefore, with the duration of marriage; the value obtained using the preceding formula is a mean equal to

$$\phi' = \frac{\int\limits_0^\infty \phi'(\zeta)F(x_r + \zeta)d\zeta}{\int\limits_0^\infty F(x_r + \zeta)d\zeta}. \tag{21}$$

One could determine the age to which Eq. (21) corresponds only if one knew approximately how ϕ' decreases. This calculation is simple if ϕ' varies linearly.

The foregoing relates to the estimation of ϕ', i.e. of a quantity that depends on both the quantities ϕ and g. It is natural to seek information on these as well.

ESTIMATION OF FECUNDABILITY

Except at the beginning of marriage, estimation of fecundability is very difficult in view of our ignorance regarding the duration of nonsusceptibility after pregnancy. We cannot, therefore, easily estimate the fecundability of women other than the newly married, and it is unknown whether the fecundability of women who are already mothers is different from that of newlyweds. We know, nevertheless, that in completed families of a given size, e.g. 12 children, the mean interval between births scarcely varies until the second last [in this case that means that if the interval from marriage to the first birth is designated as I_0, the mean durations $I_1, I_2, \ldots, I_9$ are approximately equal while I_{10} and I_{11} show some increase in length]. Since a fortuitous compensation seems unlikely, there is reason to think that between the first birth and the second last birth (that is, as long as the woman is young enough) the values of the various factors determining the spacing of births, including fecundability, are constant. There is no reason why the first birth should be associated with more variation than subsequent births. Until proof to the contrary, we will assume, therefore, that the fecundability of a married woman remains for years almost at the same level as at marriage.

THE DISCRETE CASE: GINI'S METHOD

To study the fecundability of newlyweds, it is preferable to abandon the continuous notation used until now. Let p be the probability of conception in the course of a menstrual cycle, where the cycle is assumed to be of a fixed duration equal to one month. Let us consider, then, a homogeneous group with fecundability p in which the couples were married on the same date and had no premarital conceptions. If the original number is put equal to unity, there are p conceptions expected the first month, $p(1-p)$ the second, $p(1-p)^2$ the third, and so on.

In heterogeneous groups characterized by a density $f(p)$, the expected number of conceptions in the first month is $\bar{p}$ and in the second month it is $\bar{p}-\bar{p}^2(1+c^2)$, where c is the coefficient of variation of p [c is equal to the standard deviation divided by the mean]. The complement of the ratio of the second month's conceptions to those of the first is expected to be $1-\left[\dfrac{\bar{p}-\bar{p}^2(1+c^2)}{\bar{p}}\right]$ $= \bar{p}(1+c^2)$. This is the same as the mean fecundability of women conceiving the first month, which may be written as:

$$\int p \, \frac{pf(p)}{\bar{p}} \, dp = \bar{p}(1 + c^2). \qquad (22)$$

More generally, the complement of the ratio of the expected conceptions of the $(n+1)$th month to those of the nth month is equal to the mean fecundability of women conceiving in the nth month. The mean fecundability of women conceiving in the course of the first n months of marriage is equal to a weighted mean of the preceding quantities, the weights being the number of women conceiving the first, second, . . . , nth month, i.e. the denominators of the preceding quantities. It is written:

$$\sum_{i=0}^{i=n-1} \frac{\int p \cdot p(1-p)^i f(p) dp}{\int p(1-p)^i f(p) dp} \times \frac{\int p(1-p)^i f(p) dp}{\sum_{0}^{n-1} \int p(1-p)^i f(p) dp} . \tag{23}$$

As n increases indefinitely, this quantity approaches $\bar{p}$, which is thus the mean fecundability of women who conceive at least once.

The essentials of this theory are due to C. Gini. Gini proposed, as an index, the mean fecundability during the early months of marriage, with the exception of the first month because, he says, the assumption on which the theory rests is not valid for the first month: "fecundability being lower in the first month than in the second due to the frequent virginity of the wife," and because "early abortions are especially frequent in products of conception of the first month because of honeymoon trips and perhaps other circumstances." (Gini, [1], p. 889–892.)

We will not dispute that the first month of marriage plays a somewhat special role; besides, since the date of marriage is often chosen in relation to the menses, this may affect the probability of conception in the first month. These theoretical difficulties, however, seem to have no great practical significance. Accordingly, we will assume, failing proof to the contrary, that the assumptions hold from the beginning of marriage.

In any case, the indices advocated by C. Gini present a very great advantage in that they avoid the effects of many disturbing influences. One can assume that the first months of marriage are all affected to the same extent by these diverse causes: mortality, migration and even errors or omissions in records of first births. If it causes complete sterility, limitation of births itself, temporary or permanent, should not play more than a negligible role since, in the very first months of marriage, there is unlikely to be appreciable variation in the proportion of couples who adopt or abandon contraceptive practice.

In fact, since contraceptive measures are not completely effective, couples who use them are considered to be slightly fecund rather than sterile. At the time of marriage, the number of such couples may be sufficiently large to affect appreciably the fecundability of women conceiving in the first months of marriage. Hence, even if one wishes to estimate only the "natural" fecundability of women conceiving in one or a few of the first months of marriage, it is necessary to work with data from noncontracepting populations, or at least from populations using little contraception. This requirement is even more imperative for an estimate of the mean fecundability of newlyweds.

In this latter case one ought, moreover, to take into account the progression of sterility. But since women generally marry young, its influence can in practice be considered negligible.

A more serious difficulty arises from premarital conceptions. These may result from the fact that in certain populations sexual relations generally begin before marriage. In this case, women not pregnant at marriage are a selected group with low fecundability; whatever method is used, we will therefore succeed only in measuring the fecundability of a nonrepresentative sample. In this case, the fecundability of newlyweds is as difficult to measure as that of women who are already mothers.

Let us return to our formulas. If the mean fecundability of women conceiving in the first month is $\bar{p}(1+c^2)$, then its ratio to that of nonpregnant fecund newlyweds, $\bar{p}$, is equal to $1+c^2$; we therefore have an estimate of c^2, and hence an idea of the dispersion of fecundability. If we assume, as does Gini, that the first month of marriage is a special case, we can apply the same formulas to the fecund women conceiving after the first month of marriage and determine their mean fecundability and its coefficient of variation; it is less than that of the whole group since the conceptions of the first month remove from observation a greater proportion of women of high fecundability than of low fecundability.

INTERVALS BETWEEN BIRTHS

We have already seen that in the case of a homogeneous group (ϕ, g), the mean interval between births is $g+1/\phi$; by a change of origin we have equated marriage to a birth; if one returns to the real origin at marriage, the mean interval between marriage and the first birth is reduced by $g-g_0$ and becomes g_0+1/ϕ.

In discrete notation, the mean number of ovulations (or of months) between marriage and the first conception is equal to $p+2p(1-p)+\ldots+np(1-p)^{n-1}$, that is, on setting $1-p=q$,

$$p\frac{d}{dq}\left[\sum_{i=1}^{\infty} q^i\right] = p\frac{d}{dq}\left[\frac{q}{1-q}\right] = \frac{1}{p}. \qquad (24)$$

If k is the mean interval, counted in menstrual cycles (or months), between marriage and the first ovulation, the mean interval between marriage and first conception is equal to $(k-1) + \dfrac{1}{p}$. If we assume k equal to $1/2$, the mean interval is $1/p - 1/2$. Division by 13 (or by 12) gives the mean interval in years; on adding g_0 we have the interval between marriage and the first live birth.

In a heterogeneous group the mean interval, $\bar{\imath}$, between births is given, in the continuous case, by the relation

$$\bar{\imath} = \int\int (g + 1/\phi)f(\phi)h(g)d\phi dg = \bar{g} + 1/\bar{\phi}_h. \tag{25}$$

One can also write, since $i = 1/\phi'$,

$$\bar{\imath} = \int \frac{k(\phi')d\phi'}{\phi'} = \frac{1}{\bar{\phi}'_h} \tag{26}$$

Since $\bar{\phi}_h' < \bar{\phi}'$, it follows that $1/\bar{\imath} < \bar{\phi}'$, $\bar{\imath} > 1/\bar{\phi}'$. Analogous relations hold in the discrete case. In particular, the mean interval between marriage and the first conception is equal to $k-1+(1/\bar{p}_h)$. Evidently, $\bar{p}_h < \bar{p}$; but, the inverse of the mean interval to conception, equal to $\dfrac{\bar{p}_h}{1-(1-k)\bar{p}_h}$ is also greater than $\bar{p}_h$. In practice the difference between $\bar{p}_h$ and $\bar{p}$ is generally expected to be large; the inverse of the mean interval must therefore be less than $\bar{p}$.

The foregoing holds in the absence of sterility; its presence may modify the mean intervals between births. Let $n(x)dx$ be the births of a given order that would occur in $(x, x+dx)$ after the preceding birth in the absence of sterility, and let $F'(x)$ be the proportion of couples still fecund x years after the preceding birth, when all were, by definition, fecund. The mean interval between births becomes

$$\bar{\imath}' = \frac{\int xn(x)F'(x)dx}{\int n(x)F'(x)dx}. \tag{27}$$

This is a new weighted mean of x with larger weights for low values of x and smaller weights for high values; $\bar{\imath}'$ is therefore smaller than $\bar{\imath}$; its inverse is consequently larger than that of $\bar{\imath}$. One then wishes to determine whether $1/\bar{\imath}'$ can equal or surpass $\bar{\phi}'$. For a homogeneous group of medium or high fecundability, the reduction in the mean interval by sterility at younger ages, and even up to about 40 years, is almost negligible. The reduction at older ages, on the contrary, may be very great with low and very low values of fecundability.

From the little we know of the distribution of fecundability, its mean is sufficiently high so that sterility will not affect the interval between births until older ages. However, the dispersion of fecundability is apparently great. Hence, those with low fecundability, although probably small in number, may have a sufficient effect to reduce the mean interval appreciably.

From available information on the mean interval between marriage and the first birth by the woman's age, there does not appear to be a reduction with increasing age. No doubt these data relate to populations that already practice contraception and should be verified. We think, however, we may assume that, except at older ages, the reduction in the mean interval to the first birth caused by the onset of sterility is not very important. It follows that $\bar{i}' \approx \bar{i}$, and therefore, the inverse of the mean interval between marriage and the first birth, $1/\bar{i}_1'$ will be less than ϕ, given that age at marriage is still low. If $\bar{i}'$ is the mean interval between two births calculated for relatively low ages (the first and the second birth for example), $1/\bar{i}'$ should, for the same reasons, be less than ϕ'.

Instead of the mean interval between two births of a given order, we could calculate the mean interval between all births. Let us examine what would happen in this case. Consider women who marry young; let x be the duration of marriage and dS the risk of sterility between x and $x + dx$. When age at marriage is low, $\dfrac{dS}{dx}$ is negligible when x is low; when $\dfrac{dS}{dx}$ is not negligible, x is large enough so that cumulative fertility is approximately equal to $\phi'x$ for a homogeneous group of fertility ϕ'.

Let us pass to the calculation of intervals. For women who will become sterile at x, let ζ be the duration of marriage at a given birth. In the interval $(\zeta, \zeta+d\zeta)$, there are $\phi' d\zeta$ births (except when ζ is low, which is unimportant for what follows). If ζ is between 0 and $x-g$, then $\phi' e^{-\phi(x-\zeta-g)} d\zeta$ of these children are last births. If ζ is between $x-g$ and x, all $\phi' d\zeta$ births are last births. The mean duration of marriage at the last childbirth is, therefore,

$$\left(x - \frac{g}{2}\right) \phi' g + \int_0^{x-g} \phi' \zeta e^{-\phi(x-\zeta-g)} d\zeta \; ; \qquad (28)$$

that is,

$$\phi' \left[g\left(x - \frac{g}{2} \right) + \frac{x-g}{\phi} - \frac{1}{\phi^2} + \frac{e^{-\phi(x-g)}}{\phi^2} \right], \qquad (29)$$

or, ignoring the term in $e^{-\phi(x-g)}$,

$$\phi' \left[(x-g)\left(g + \frac{1}{\phi} \right) + \frac{g^2}{2} - \frac{1}{\phi^2} \right] = x-g + \phi'\left(\frac{g^2}{2} - \frac{1}{\phi^2} \right). \tag{30}$$

The duration of marriage at first birth is equal to

$$\int_{g_0}^{x} \zeta\phi e^{-\phi(\zeta-g_0)}\,d\zeta,$$

which is

$$(g_0 + 1/\phi)(1 - e^{-\phi(x-g_0)}) - (x - g_0)e^{-\phi(x-g_0)}, \tag{31}$$

which, for sufficiently large x, reduces to $g_0 + 1/\phi$. Then, the time between first and last births reduces to $x - g - g_0 - 1/\phi + \phi'(g^2/2 - 1/\phi^2)$. The number of births of order 2 and higher is, on the other hand, equal to

$$\phi'x - 1 + e^{-\phi(x-g_0)} \tag{32}$$

being, for all practical purposes, $\phi'x-1$. For a heterogeneous group, the time between first and last births is equal to $x-k$, where

$$k = \int\int \left[g + g_0 + \frac{1}{\phi} - \phi'\left(\frac{g^2}{2} - \frac{1}{\phi^2} \right) \right] f(\phi)h(g)d\phi dg. \tag{33}$$

The total number of births is $\bar{\phi}'x-1$. For all values of x, one then has $\int(\phi'x-1)dS = \phi'\int xdS - \int dS$ births and, for the durations: $\int xdS - k\int dS$. In practice, only large values of x enter the picture. Therefore, the ratio of births to durations is in practice reduced to $\bar{\phi}'$. We emphasize, however, that this result is valid only for the assumptions made; in particular that the population is noncontracepting and that the distribution of fecundability is such that the frequency of low values (those for which $e^{-\phi x}$ and $xe^{-\phi x}$ are not negligible) is negligible.

METHOD OF THE DURATION
OF EXPOSURE TO RISK

Let us begin with the relatively simple case of first births. Investigations have been performed to determine the interval be-

tween marriage and the first conception in women without premarital conceptions who did not use contraceptives; this period
is the duration of exposure to the risk of conception. For example, this was done in Pearl's study (Pearl [1]) of women who
had just given birth, in the study by Stix and Notestein [1] in
cooperation with the consultants of a birth control clinic and
in that by Whelpton and Kiser [1] of couples in Indianapolis. In
the case of a study of couples married for some time, such as in
Indianapolis, the mean duration of exposure to risk of noncontracepting couples is comparable to the mean interval between
marriage and the first conception as studied in the preceding
pages. In the other studies, the survey included women with
varying durations of marriage, and there is no assurance that the
distribution of the subjects by duration of marriage at the first
conception resembles what would be observed in a well-defined
group of women whose history could be followed from the beginning of marriage.

Thus in Pearl's study, the proportion of women with a long
duration of marriage at the time of the study may have been
very low because of the increase in the number of marriages associated with the growth of the United States population and
perhaps also because deliveries at hospitals were less frequent
in the older generations. The study of Stix and Notestein carried
an even greater risk of selection. It is probable that married
women with a long interval between marriage and the first birth
and, therefore, with low fecundability, did not on the average
attend birth control clinics as frequently as did women with a
first birth soon after marriage.

Now, in calculating a mean, large values affect the result considerably. The effect of the selection mentioned above may, therefore, be sufficient to make the mean duration of exposure quite
different from what one would find in working with a well-
defined marriage cohort observed from marriage.

Actually, the results from Pearl's study and the Indianapolis
study show no marked difference in the interval between marriage and the first conception among couples who were noncontracepting before the first birth. In the first case, the interval was
10.9 months for white women (Pearl [1], p. 333, Table XV), as
compared with 11.4 months in Indianapolis (Whelpton and Kiser
[1], Chap. VIII, p. 342). On the other hand, Stix and Notestein
([1], p. 34) observed a mean of 4.3 months. From the Indianapolis

data, it is possible to estimate the proportion of women conceiving during the first month.[4] This proportion is about 20 percent, although the inverse of the mean duration is approximately 9 percent. These results conform with the theory and illustrate its value. They show to what degree fecundability may be underestimated by equating it to the inverse of the interval from marriage to the first conception. This underestimation is due to differences in fecundability between women. The group of women here appears to be very heterogeneous. Thus, it is not surprising that when selection operates, significantly inconsistent results are obtained. Such selection must explain the results obtained by Stix and Notestein, among others.

After the first birth, the reports use different methods of computing the duration of exposure to risk. This risk does not reappear immediately after delivery; for some women who are nonsusceptible during lactation, it may reappear only after several months. However, Pearl allows only ten days; the other authors, one month. It is obvious that in this way one can obtain only a hypothetical mean duration of exposure to risk. We prefer simply to give average intervals between births obtained by adding the durations of pregnancy and of nonsusceptibility assumed by each author to the mean durations of exposure to risk.

In the Indianapolis survey (Whelpton and Kiser [1], Chap. VIII, pp. 348 and 352, Tables C and D), the mean intervals between the first and second conceptions and between the second and third conceptions are about twenty-seven months; Stix and Notestein ([1], p. 32, Table 9) give a little more than twenty months as the mean for all intervals between births; Pearl's ([1], p. 333, estimate from data in Table XV and XVI) corresponding value is about twenty-six months. The absolute values of the differences between the different studies are about the same as for the differences for first conceptions. Relative to the mean intervals between births, however, the differences are less impressive because gestation and the postpartum nonsusceptible period are added to the interval between births.

For Indianapolis, the mean interval, which takes into account only births of low order, should, according to the theory (see pp. 18–19), be greater than the inverse of the mean natural fertility of the population in question, though some long intervals may

---

[4] The proportion conceiving before one and one-half months of marriage is given.

have been missed because the duration of observation was limited. In the other cases, all births are included. For noncontracepting populations, the inverse of the mean interval should have been close to ϕ'. But the populations studied are definitely contraceptors. The data for estimating intervals between births were obtained from noncontracepting couples who remained such only as long as their family size was fairly limited. Therefore, in the data for intervals between births, lower order intervals [and, therefore, long intervals], receive more weight than they would in a noncontracepting population. Thus, the inverse of the mean interval is still below the natural fertility of the groups studied (but doubtless less so than in the Indianapolis case) to the degree that disturbing causes mentioned above do not bias the results too much. For the women studied by Stix and Notestein, it is then obvious that the group is highly selected.

PEARL'S PREGNANCY RATE AND LIVE BIRTH RATE

The procedure just described amonts to estimating natural fertility by computing the mean duration of exposure to risk per conception, and taking the inverse of this mean duration. In this case, the mean duration is computed as the total duration of exposure to risk for all the women, divided by the total number of conceptions. Pearl, however, did not limit himself to this procedure [which we shall call Pearl's rate I]. He also calculated, for each woman, another pregnancy rate or live birth rate by taking, for example, either the inverse of the duration between marriage and the first conception or else by dividing the number of conceptions or live births by the duration of exposure to risk. He then averaged the rates thus obtained. [We shall call this Pearl's rate II.] Let us confine ourselves to the case of primiparae and see where Pearl's procedure leads.

We shall use the discrete model and begin with a homogeneous group of fecundability p. The women conceiving the first month would be assigned a rate of one, those conceiving the second month, a rate of $1/2$ and so on. Since the probability of conceiving in the first month is p, in the second month, $p(1-p)$, etc. the expected value of Pearl's rate II is equal to:

$$p + \frac{p(1-p)}{2} + \frac{p(1-p)^2}{3} + \ldots + \frac{p(1-p)^{n-1}}{n} + \ldots$$

which is equal to p if $p = 1$, and to

$$\frac{p}{1-p}\left[\sum_{i=1}^{\infty}\frac{(1-p)^i}{i}\right] = \frac{p}{1-p}\,\text{Log}\,1/p, \qquad (34)$$

if $p < 1$, which is greater than p. For average values of p (about 20 percent), the relative difference is large since the mean pregnancy rate in Eq. (34) is equal to 40 percent. For smaller values of p, the relative difference is even greater. Thus for $p = 2$ percent, the rate is 8 percent. For a heterogeneous group, Pearl's mean rate II is equal to the mean of the expected rates of the component homogeneous groups; i.e. an average of values that are all larger than p. Therefore, this mean is larger than $\bar{p}$.

We have seen that the mean durations of exposure to risk between marriage and the first conception were similar in Pearl's study and in the Indianapolis survey. Therefore, it seems legitimate to attribute the same mean fecundability, i.e. 21 percent, to the women in these studies.

Pearl's report ([1], Tables XVII, XX, and XXI) gives much higher mean pregnancy rates (28 percent for white women). Here, only women without gynecological abnormalities, i.e. selected cases, are included, but chiefly, the computation was done according to the method just described.

Pearl's rate I from Table XVI in the same book is 9 percent. The average fecundability must be about 20 percent. The average pregnancy rate II is 28 percent. The order of the three figures is as expected from theory. Undoubtedly the spread between the last two may be a bit exaggerated by the selection of women without gynecological abnormalities. Still, since we know that the difference between the mean fecundability and Pearl's rate II may be appreciable, it is not proven that the observed difference is due to selection.

Let us say, in any case, that the difference between the methods of computation can explain the differences between the three results: 9, 20, and 28 percent.

CONCLUSION

The example just given shows that preliminary investigation of indices is not irrelevant. For lack of such study, Pearl's book, referred to previously, is full of pitfalls; the reader who is able to overcome them nevertheless remains puzzled when confronted by very different values which appear, at first sight, to be estimates of the same quantity.

The confusion itself, rather than the use of one index rather than another, is regrettable. In demography the adoption of an index may be governed by many considerations, among which simplicity and convenience are important.

In this regard, the mean duration of exposure to risk per conception, or per live birth, has advantages as soon as the major errors cited are eliminated. The fact that the mean nonsusceptible period after delivery intervenes here is especially interesting. In fact, if we assume, as appears reasonable, that the first pregnancy does not modify fecundability more than subsequent pregnancies do, the difference between the mean duration of exposure to risk: (a) between marriage and the first conception and (b) between a delivery and the next conception, is equal to the mean duration of nonsusceptibility after each delivery. For Indianapolis, the difference is about seven months.

Confusion begins when, for this mean duration, its inverse is substituted. One is then faced with an index named "the average number of conceptions per year of exposure to risk" or, if the duration of pregnancy is added, "the number of conceptions per year of marriage among fecund couples," i.e. an index which by its name is indistinguishable from ϕ' Therefore, we must not be surprised that it was used in place of ϕ'.

Our investigation has shown that since populations are very heterogeneous for ϕ and g, one should not, in calculating the natural cumulative fertility, estimate ϕ' as the inverse of the mean interval between births deduced from the mean duration of exposure to risk of not yet contracepting fertile couples.

To compute the expected number of births, given natural fertility of couples remaining fecund for x years, it is necessary to estimate ϕ'. However, estimates of ϕ' must almost always be confined to noncontracepting populations, since the computation requires the natural fertility of couples who have already been married a long time. Lacking data on a noncontracepting population, ϕ' might be computed for couples who have never used contraception, provided that this does not select couples of low fecundity, as is to be expected.

On the other hand, the mean duration of exposure to risk may be computed from data on couples who are not yet contraceptors although they will be so later. Unfortunately such data are not available. We would need data about the distributions of ϕ and g, but, under the most favorable circumstances, we know only the means $\bar{\phi}$ and $\bar{g}$ and the coefficient of variation c of ϕ.

In other words, in the present state of knowledge, it is difficult to say, from the natural mean interval between low order births, how many children may be expected, on the average, during x years of fecund marriage among the couples in the population whose mean interval has been observed.

Outside of research on ϕ and g, which would certainly be difficult, investigations of noncontracepting populations might be performed, which might empirically show a relation between $\bar{\phi}'$ and $\bar{\imath}$, and permit us to determine $\bar{\phi}'$ from a knowledge of $\bar{\imath}$. Assuming that $\bar{\phi}'$ could thus be estimated in this way, there would remain the problem of combining it with the proportion F of married, fecund women at each age, the estimation of which is difficult itself.

In a nutshell, many obstacles hamper the study of natural fertility and its components. Much work still remains to be done in this area.

CHAPTER TWO

Fertility and Family:
Mathematical Models I*

EDITORS' SUMMARY

Having pursued his investigations further, M. Henry shows in this paper (published in 1957) that it is misleading to ignore the differentiation between various pregnancy outcomes. Here he therefore adds to his models explicit provision for two kinds of outcomes: a live birth and pregnancy wastage. He postulates two distinct distributions of the duration of the nonsusceptible period, one for each outcome of pregnancy. The investigation is limited to homogeneous groups of fecund women, but fecundability and the probability that a pregnancy ends in live birth, as well as the distribution of the duration of nonsusceptibility, are assumed to depend on the woman's age. Models are formulated in both continuous and discrete time. The relation between these three functions of age (fecundability, the probability of fetal loss and the mean duration of nonsusceptibility) and resultant conception rates and fertility rates is the principal subject of study. Numerical illustrations of the model are given, with hypothetical values for the parameters.

---

*Originally printed in French as "Fécondité et famille. Modèles mathématiques (I)." *Population* 12, no. 3 (Juil-Sept. 1957): 413–444.

CONTENTS

INTRODUCTION

We may expect that investigations of fertility will increasingly make use of case histories of families established from surveys or reconstituted from documents. We are realizing that it is desirable to take into account an increasing number of aspects of fertility. Since each one of these is an element in the family history, it is reasonable that we attempt to know this history in its entirety and that we do not limit ourselves to any one aspect, which may in the end be completely devoid of interest. The examination of all the numerical data in these case histories makes it possible to investigate fertility and the process of family building from many angles, and to derive a large number of results.

This very profusion of indices is, however, a source of difficulties. First of all, for presentation: we cannot abstain from classifying the data, but the choice of classification may be completely arbitrary if essential relations between various results are not known. The interpretation of the results is even more hazardous without sufficient knowledge of the relations between different facets that the observations may present.

Recourse to mathematical models is one means of dealing with this uncomfortable situation. A model that allows us to express any observation in terms of a few fundamental functions provides insights into the significance and interrelations of observed data. The presentation of the findings may be facilitated. Interpretation definitely acquires a solid basis which was previously lacking.

Although justified in principle, recourse to models may never-

SUMMARY OF NOTATION

For simplicity of presentation, we treat the total number as equal to unity and refer to various expected rates or densities as the number of occurrences.

x or ζ — Age of the woman.

x_o — Age of the woman at marriage.

p — Fecundability or probability that a married woman will conceive per unit time outside of non-susceptible periods.

v — Proportion of conceptions terminating in live births.

g — Duration of nonsusceptibility.

$\bar{g}$ — Mean duration of nonsusceptibility.

$\bar{g}_a$ and $\bar{g}_v$ — Mean duration of nonsusceptibility respectively corresponding to conceptions ending in abortion or live birth.

G — Upper limit of the duration of nonsusceptibility following conception.

g_o — Duration of a pregnancy that terminates in a live birth.

σ_g^2 — Variance of g.

$K(\zeta,g)$ — Probability that a woman who conceived at age ζ is still not susceptible at age $\zeta + g$.

$K_a(\zeta,g)$ and $K_v(\zeta,g)$ — Corresponding probabilities respectively for conceptions ending in abortion and live birth.

$h(g)$ — Probability density of g (p.d.f. of g).

$C(x)dx$ — Expected number of conceptions in the age interval $(x, x + dx)$ or total fertility rate.

$Z(x) = C_2(x) - C_1(x)$ — Difference between two instantaneous total fertility rates, corresponding respectively to marriage at age x_2 and x_1, where $x_2 > x_1$.

$B(x)dx$ — Expected number of live births in the age interval $(x, x + dx)$, or effective fertility rate.

$V(x)dx$ — Expected number of conceptions in $(x, x + dx)$ terminating in live births.

$p(x)dx$ Fecundability or probability of conceiving in the interval $(x, x + dx)$.

$v(x)$ Probability that a conception occurring at age x terminates in a live birth.

$\pi(x)$ Effective fecundability, i.e. $[v(x)p(x)]$.

$D(x)$ Difference between $V_1(x)$ and $V_2(x)$, i.e. error made when $V_2(x)$, the solution to Eq. (29), is used to measure conceptions terminating in live births as an approximation to $V_1(x)$, the solution to Eq. (18).

$Q(x)$ Cumulative mean number of conceptions by age x for a woman married at age x_0.

$E(x)$ Cumulative mean number of live births by age x or cumulative fertility by age x.

$f(x)$ Reference fertility, see Eq. (4).

For the discrete case, the same symbols are used with a subscript.

theless encounter difficulties that cast doubts on the practical value of this form of research. These doubts would be confirmed if it turned out that the models were an onerous means of arriving at intuitive results. Nevertheless, even in this case, the use of models would still be justified since we cannot know the results in advance. Also, it is reasonable to think that the difficulty of a model results from the very complexity of the phenomenon being investigated. Consequently, it seems unlikely that the relations between the different aspects of such a phenomenon can be solved intuitively or merely through skilled manipulation of statistics.

Moreover, our method of procedure will minimize the risk of useless efforts. Generally we will first investigate simplified models. If we derive important results, we will be encouraged to proceed further in research that has proven fruitful.

Several years ago we began with a very simple model (Henry, [2]) that did not explicitly provide for pregnancy wastage. Subsequently, particularly when studing the fertility of historical European populations, we became aware of the limitations of this model and were motivated to consider less restricted models. As in the previous investigation, we are concerned only with fertility in the absence of birth control. Not that we intend always to limit ourselves to this area alone, but there is no point in formulating models of fertility that include birth control without previous investigation of models without birth control.

Besides, the numerous aspects of fertility cannot all be examined within one article. These few pages are therefore merely intended:

1. to indicate the bases on which the models have been constructed.
2. to examine the relations between the legitimate fertility rate of a homogeneous group, in the absence of birth control, and the fundamental functions included in the models.

Other aspects, in particular that of family building (number of children and intervals between births), will be considered later.

BASIS OF MODELS

Underlying mathematical models of legitimate fertility and family formation are three generally accepted facts:

1. conception is impossible during pregnancy and probably also during a variable interval of time after delivery.
2. even without contraceptives, sexual relations are not always followed by conception and, vice versa, contraceptives do not always prevent conception; conception must be considered to be affected by chance.
3. conception does not always terminate in a live birth.

In order to take these facts into account, we must consider that fertility depends on three fundamental factors:

1. the duration of nonsusceptibility (g) after each conception, which depends on the duration of pregnancy and the delay in the resumption of ovulation after delivery. [We assume implicitly that sexual relations are resumed before the end of the nonsusceptible period.]
2. fecundability, or the probability (p) per unit time that a married woman will conceive outside of the periods of nonsusceptibility after conception. The unit of time may be assumed to be finite, i.e. as the mean duration of the menstrual cycle, or it may be treated as infinitely small. Hence we may formulate two types of models, one discrete and the other continuous, the former being more convenient for numerical calculations.

3. the proportion of conceptions terminating in live births (v).

Since no population is either physically or psychologically homogeneous, the fundamental factors certainly vary between different couples. Therefore it is necessary to construct models for heterogeneous groups. However, since a heterogeneous group is made up of homogeneous subgroups, we must start by studying the latter. In this article, we discuss only homogeneous groups.

For a given woman, and consequently for a homogeneous group, the duration of nonsusceptibility, g, may vary appreciably between one conception and the next, depending on whether the pregnancy did or did not reach its term, on whether the child lived or died very young, on whether nursing lasted a long or a short time, and on whether delivery did or did not cause temporary pathological sterility. Hence g must be considered a random variable with a specified distribution. The most useful way of characterizing such a distribution, for our purposes, is by the probability of still being unable to conceive at the end of a time g following the preceding conception. This probability is denoted by the symbol K_g.

A priori, K_g or p or v may be a function of several variables, including the woman's age and parity. In some of the historical or underdeveloped populations that have been studied in detail, observed fertility at any specified age is practically independent of age at marriage when the duration of marriage exceeds a few years. In contrast, there is a marked relationship between age at marriage and age-specific fertility in populations that practice birth control widely. The absence of this relation in populations that are ignorant of or little inclined to practice birth control, leads us to assume that in the case of natural fertility, the fundamental functions K_g, p and v are functions of a single variable, the woman's age. This is no longer true when birth control is practiced. In that case, the probability of conception depends on contraceptive practice, which is itself influenced by the number of children already born. In short, there may be two distinct types of models according to whether the fundamental functions depend only on the woman's age or on her age and parity. As already stated, we are concerned here only with the case without birth control.

In this case, all aspects of fertility and of the constitution of the family in a homogeneous group depend on three functions of the woman's age: K_g, the probability of still being unable to conceive after an interval g since the preceding conception; p, fecundability or the probability of conception per unit time outside of the periods of nonsusceptibility following conception; and v, the proportion of conceptions ending in live births.

FERTILITY

The legitimate fertility rate is the most current term for the fertility of married women.[1] The investigation mentioned earlier (Henry, [2]), of the simplest model (constant fecundability, invariant duration of nonsusceptibility, equating conception to live birth) has already shown that the relation between the expected legitimate fertility rate and the fundamental functions is, at first sight, complex: The fertility rate is the sum of a constant plus an oscillating function which becomes damped with increasing duration of marriage. The oscillating function depends on the initial conditions and would be zero only in a hypothetical case never occurring in practice [i.e. if the nonsusceptible period did not exist. See Chapter One, p. 7] Nevertheless, if we disregard the oscillations, the relation is simple because the nonoscillatory term of the fertility rate is constant, as are the fundamental factors.

Since the oscillations are the unavoidable consequence of the existence of temporary nonsusceptible periods following each conception, we must also expect to find them in more complicated models. On the other hand, we cannot predict whether fertility will still have a simple relation to the fundamental functions outside of these oscillations. Let us illustrate this point by an example: suppose that we can define an "aptitude for procreation" on the basis of the fundamental functions. Suppose also that this aptitude reaches a unique maximum at, for example, the age of 20. If it were possible to eliminate the oscillations from the expected fertility rate, would this rate also have a unique maximum? If so, is this maximum reached at, before, or after the age of 20? In other words, does the curve of the legitimate fertility rate according to the woman's age closely follow the curve of the aptitude for procreation, or is there an appreciable discrepancy between the two? The interpretation of the results of current studies of legitimate natural fertility, i.e. the series of fertility

---

[1] Strictly speaking, it should be called the fertility of married couples, but since this is an awkward term, it is easier to use the term the fertility of married women as a substitute.

rates by age or by age group, depends on the answer to this question.

The foregoing is only one example of the problems of interpreting data. In general, we obtain data on fertility of one or more groups. Observing differences by age in the same group or differences between groups, we would like to know what inferences we can make regarding the fundamental functions at different ages or in different groups. [The purpose of this paper is to explore these questions by starting with certain assumptions about the fundamental functions and seeing how they are reflected in the fertility rate.]

FUNDAMENTAL RELATIONS

Using the notation defined at the beginning, the number of conceptions in the interval $(x, x+dx)$ is equal to the product of $p(x)dx$ by the number of susceptible women, i.e. the total number of women in the group (taken as equal to unity) minus the number still nonsusceptible following the preceding conception. We therefore write, suppressing dx on both sides of the equation:

$$C(x) = p(x)[1 - \int_0^G C(x-g)K(x-g,g)dg]. \qquad (1)$$

For women marrying at age x_0, this equation holds starting from age x_0 if $C(x)$ is known in the interval (x_0-G, x_0). If there have been no premarital conceptions, $C(x)$ is zero for $x < x_0$.

In our homogeneous group, consider two sub-groups of women, one of which married at age x_1 and the other at age x_2; designate their instantaneous total fertility as $C_1(x)$ and $C_2(x)$ respectively. Equation (1) holds equally for $C_1(x)$ and $C_2(x)$ after the higher age x_2. If the difference, $C_2(x)-C_1(x)$, is denoted by $Z(x)$, we write:

$$Z(x) = -p(x) \int_0^G Z(x-g)K(x-g,g)dg. \qquad (2)$$

From this equation, it is clear that $Z(x)$ cannot have the same sign for a period of time greater than G. $Z(x)$ is therefore alternately positive and negative; on the other hand, if $Z(x)$ is zero for a given value X of x, its sign must change at least once in the interval $(X-G,X)$.[2]

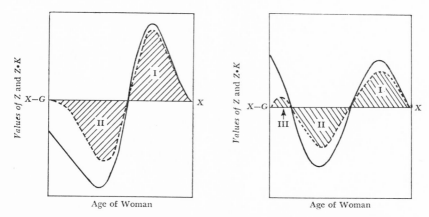

Figure 1 (Left), Figure 2 (Right). Schematic diagram of $Z(x)$ and $Z(x)K(g)$. In each case, the solid line represents $Z(x-g)$ while the broken line represents the product $Z(x-g)K(x-g, g)$. In Figure 1, $Z(x)$ has one zero in $(X-G,X)$; in Figure 2, it has two zeros in this interval of time.

$Z(x)$ may have an odd or an even number of zeros in the interval $(X-G,X)$; with one or two zeros for example, we obtain Figures 1 and 2 respectively. Since $K \leqq 1$, the curve representing the product ZK lies between the curve representing Z and the x-axis. When $Z(x)$ is zero, Eq. (2) shows that the algebraic sum of the shaded areas lying between the x-axis, the curve ZK, and the verticals at $X-G$ and X, is zero, This area is the algebraic sum of the shaded loops I and II (Fig. 1) or I, II and III (Fig. 2). When the distribution of the duration of nonsusceptibility does not vary with the woman's age, K depends on g only, decreasing as g increases. This is also true when the distribution is shifted or skewed to the right with increasing age in such a manner that for all g, $K(x-g,g)$ decreases as g increases. In both cases, the area of the loops formed by Z decreases in absolute value from one loop to the next with increasing age; at the limit, this surface is zero.

On the other hand, from the figures alone, we cannot say that the absolute value of the area of the loops decreases from left to right if $K(x-g,g)$ does not decrease constantly with increasing g.

[2] The functions C are continuous beginning with marriage; therefore Z is also continuous. The only discontinuous change of sign is that which may occur at x_0 if the values selected in the interval (x_0-G,x_0) are such that the difference between $C(x_0-\varepsilon)$ and $C(x_0+\varepsilon)$ is not infinitely small when ε is infinitely small.

This situation could occur, for example, if the distribution of nonsusceptibility shifted to the left with increasing age. This change would still have to occur rapidly; in any case, it could not last very long because the reduction possible in the mean duration of nonsusceptibility is very limited.

In conclusion, the oscillations in the function $Z(x)$ become damped with increases in either age or the duration of marriage, whether after a certain age or a certain marital duration.

The same conclusion is reached as in the simplest model: *at a given age, the instantaneous fertility rates of women from a homogeneous group married at different ages x_1 and x_2 ($x_2 > x_1$) are not equal; but their difference is a damped oscillatory function of the duration of marriage; if this duration is sufficiently long, the difference is zero.*

For heterogeneous groups, the oscillations related to the constituent homogeneous groups are superimposed; but, since they do not coincide, the result is an attenuation of the oscillations. Besides, measures of legitimate fertility are most frequently based on long time intervals (five-year age groups, for example) in which the damping is still more marked. This explains why, at the same age, fertility rates may, in practice, be independent of age at marriage, although this may not be the case in theory.

DISCRETE CASE

In the discrete case, we obtain an equation analogous to Eq. (1), written as:[3]

$$C_x = p_x \left[1 - \sum_{g=1}^{g=G} C_{x-g} K_{x-g,g} \right].$$ (3)

Equation (3), rather than Eq. (1), was used in the numerical calculations. Since ovulation is by nature a discrete event, this equation conforms better to reality, where the duration of the menstrual cycle, or even more simply the month, is taken as the unit of time.

---

[3] In the discrete case, a woman who conceives during the ζth month and remains sterile for g months is able to conceive again starting with month $\zeta+g+1$. If $h(g)$ is the probability that the duration of nonsusceptibility is equal to g, the proportion K_g of women who are still unable to conceive during month $\zeta+g$ is equal to $h(g)+\ldots+h(G)$.

CENTRAL FERTILITY

From Eq. (1), $C(x)$ is the solution of an integral equation, which depends on an arbitrarily selected function in the interval $(x_0, x_0 - G)$. This function defines the initial conditions. In the discrete case, the set of Eq. (3) relative to the various C_x (from $x = x_0$ to $x = \omega$, the maximum (finite) age to be considered) forms a system of linear equations, the solutions of which depend on G arbitrary values, $C_{x_0 - G}, \ldots, C_{x_0 - 1}$, defining the initial conditions. Each of the Solutions $C_{x_0}, \ldots, C_\omega$ of this system is a linear form of the G quantities $C_{x_0 - G}, \ldots, C_{x_0 - 1}$.

Having made this point, let us return to the results of the preceding paragraphs. The difference between two solutions of Eq. (1) or (3) is of the damped oscillatory type. Strictly speaking, these are oscillations of one solution starting from a given value x_0 of x, around another solution starting from the same value. That these oscillations become damped means that the difference between two solutions tends to disappear with increasing distance from x_0. In other words, the effect of the initial conditions is reduced with the passage of time. This does not mean, however, that the common value toward which the various solutions tend is itself without oscillations; if the second order derivatives of $p(x)$ or the second order differences of p_x have a constant sign, there is not necessarily a solution $C(x)$ (or C_x) with the same property.

Nevertheless, confronted with a fertility curve presenting alternating maxima and minima (compare Figures 3 and 5) or oscillations apparent from the slope of the tangent, one would naturally attempt to find a less oscillating curve, which might be thought of as representing fertility at each age in some way, by eliminating those oscillations that we believe to be parasitic. In other words, we attempt to relate the different solutions to the one which presents the "minimum oscillation." To do this, we first define the solution giving "minimum oscillation," i.e. that solution whose derivative (or first difference, in the discrete case) varies least after the given age x_0.

In the continuous case, it is difficult to satisfy this condition. In the discrete case, it is sufficient to determine the initial values $C_{x_0 - G}, \ldots, C_{x_0 - 1}$, in such a manner that the sum of the squares of the second order differences, starting at x_0, will be a minimum. These values are the solutions of a system of G linear equations with G unknowns.

The solution that corresponds to the initial conditions so determined, will be called *the central solution relative to the age at marriage* x_o. In some circumstances, the central solution may be independent of x_o but this is not generally the case. Since we attempt, in practice, to relate the observed fertility of women married at all possible ages to a single central solution, we are led to select the central solution that corresponds to the lowest possible age at marriage. This particular central solution will be called the *central fertility rate or central fertility* [pertaining to conceptions]. We now must find out what this central fertility represents.

In the simplest case, where p and K_g do not depend on the woman's age, Eq. (1) and (3) have a constant solution equal to $p/(1+\bar{g}p)$, where $\bar{g}$ is the mean duration of nonsusceptibility. This constant solution is the central fertility;[4] it is linked to p in a very simple manner. When p varies with the woman's age, but the distribution of the duration of nonsusceptibility does not, the function:

$$f(x) = \frac{p(x)}{1 + \bar{g}p(x)} \tag{4}$$

is an analogous expression, with $p(x)$ replacing p. Then $f(x)$ may be considered to characterize the aptitude for procreation of women aged x. This function, designated as *reference fertility*, is equal to zero when p is zero and passes through an extreme at the same time as p does. Therefore, it is of interest to compare $f(x)$ with the central fertility. There is no point in doing so for all functions $p(x)$; we shall restrict ourselves to functions which may be encountered in reality.

Since a woman is fecund only during a limited range of ages, $p(x)$ must be equal to zero prior to an age α and after an age ω, the function reaches at least one maximum between α and ω, but observations do not justify an assumption of several maxima separated by intermediate minima. To explain data on the length of intervals between births in complete families of a specified size, it is sufficient for $p(x)$ to reach a maximum at an age β, remain at a plateau or drop slowly from age β to an age γ and then

---

[4] [See Eq. (44) and for a parallel result, see Eq. (5) in Chapter One, page 7.]

drop rather rapidly from age γ to age ω.[5] This is the case we will consider.

Introducing the reference fertility $f(x)$ into Eq. (1), we may write $C(x)$ as:

$$C(x) = f(x) \left[1 + \int_0^G [C(x) - C(x-g)] K(g) dg \right], \tag{5}$$

whence $C(x)$ is greater than or less than $f(x)$ depending on the sign of the difference $C(x)-C(x-g)$. Note that, from the assumption that $p(x)$ reaches a single maximum at age β, it follows that $f(x)$ reaches a single maximum at the same age β. If the central fertility $C(x)$ also presents only one maximum and if this is reached at an age β_1 (where β_1 may or may not be equal to β), then $C(x)-C(x-g)$ is positive for any value of x greater than $a+G$ and less than β_1; this difference is, in contrast, negative for any value of x greater than β_1+G. It follows that, if $C(x)$, the central fertility, like $f(x)$, the reference fertility, presents only one maximum, the central fertility is greater than the reference fertility from age $a+G$ (at least) to age β_1 and it is [lower—L.H.] from age β_1+G to age ω.

Differentiating Eq. (5) with respect to x, we obtain:

$$C'(x) = \frac{f'(x)C(x)}{f(x)} + f(x) \left[C'(x)\bar{g} - \int_0^G \frac{\partial C(x-g)}{\partial x} K(g) dg \right]. \tag{6}$$

But,[6]

$$\frac{\partial C(x-g)}{\partial x} = -\frac{\partial C(x-g)}{\partial g}, \tag{7}$$

---

[5] It is probable that not only $p(x)$ varies with age in this manner; $v(x)$ must also be [higher—L.H.] at intermediate ages than at very low or very high ages.

[6] [Equation (7) may be proved as follows:

$$\frac{\partial C(x-g)}{\partial x} = \frac{\partial C(x-g)}{\partial(x-g)} \cdot \frac{\partial(x-g)}{\partial(x)} = \frac{\partial C(x-g)}{\partial(x-g)}$$

and

$$\frac{\partial C(x-g)}{\partial g} = \frac{\partial C(x-g)}{\partial(x-g)} \cdot \frac{\partial(x-g)}{\partial g} = \frac{-\partial C(x-g)}{\partial(x-g)} \left] \right. .$$

and therefore, the integral on the extreme right hand side of Eq. (6) becomes:

$$-\int_0^G \frac{\partial C}{\partial x} K dg = \int_0^G \frac{\partial C}{\partial g} K dg = \left[\mathbf{C} \cdot \mathbf{K} \right]_0^G - \int_0^G C \frac{dK}{dg} dg. \qquad (8)$$

Defining $h(g)$ as the probability density (p.d.f.) of the duration of nonsusceptibility, we have:

$$h(g) = -\frac{dK}{dg}. \qquad (9)$$

On the other hand:

$$K(0) = 1, K(G) = 0; \qquad (10)$$

and therefore finally:

$$C'(x) = \frac{f'(x)C(x)}{f(x)} + f(x) \left[C'(x)\bar{g} - C(x) + \int_0^G C(x-g)h(g)dg \right]. \qquad (11)$$

At β_1, $C'(\beta_1)$ is zero and we therefore have:

$$\frac{f'(\beta_1)C(\beta_1)}{f(\beta_1)} = f(\beta_1) \left[C(\beta_1) - \int_0^G C(\beta_1 - g)h(g)dg \right]. \qquad (12)$$

The integral on the right hand side of Eq. (12) is a weighted mean of $C(x)$ in the interval $(\beta_1 - G, \beta_1)$; its value is lower than $C(\beta_1)$ and therefore $f'(\beta_1)$ is positive. In other words, if central fertility has a unique maximum as do the reference fertility and fecundability, it reaches this maximum at a lower age than the others, i.e. β_1 is less than β.

At age β, where $f(x)$ reaches its maximum, we have:

$$[1 - \bar{g}f(\beta)] C'(\beta) = -f(\beta) \left[C(\beta) - \int_0^G C(\beta-g)h(g)dg \right]. \qquad (13)$$

$C'(\beta)$ is negative; $C(\beta)$ therefore must be greater than the weighted mean of the quantities $C(\beta-g)$; for this to be possible, $\beta-G$ must be less than β_1 [i.e. $\beta-G < \beta_1 < \beta$].

The age when central fertility passes through a maximum is lower than the age when the reference fertility and fecundability reach their maximum, but the difference between the two ages is less than the upper limit of the duration of nonsusceptibility after each conception.

When the distribution of the duration of nonsusceptibility varies with the woman's age, various definitions of reference fertility, which need not be considered here, are possible. The case we are examining here is sufficient to show that *the curve of legitimate fertility, even neglecting the normally present disturbing oscillations, may deviate significantly from the curve of the aptitude for procreation.*

LIVE BIRTHS

Live births are related to conceptions by the equation:

$$B(x) = v(x-g_0)C(x-g_0). \tag{14}$$

Introducing $V(x)$, the rate of conceptions terminating in live births, we have:

$$V(x) = v(x)C(x). \tag{15}$$

B follows from V by a simple shift to the right by g_0.

$v(x)p(x)dx$ is the probability of a conception, in the age interval $(x, x+dx)$, that will end in a live birth. We call the quantity $v(x)p(x)$ the *effective fecundability* and designate it by $\pi(x)$. This gives us, using Eq. (1) and (15):

$$V(x) = \pi(x)\left[1 - \int_0^G V(x-g)\frac{K(x-g,g)}{v(x-g)}dg\right]. \tag{16}$$

At first glance, the instantaneous rate of effective fertility $B(x)$, which is equivalent to $V(x)$ shifted to the right, is analogous to Eq. (1). Effective fecundability $\pi(x)$ replaces the total fecundability $p(x)$, and the quantity $\dfrac{K(x-g,g)}{v(x-g)}$ replaces the probability $K(x-g,g)$. But this apparent similarity obscures a fundamental difference: $K(x-g,g)$ is a probability, whereas the quantity $\dfrac{K(x-g,g)}{v(x-g)}$, which may exceed 1, cannot be considered as such.

The duration of nonsusceptibility after conception varies greatly depending on whether conception does or does not terminate in live birth; it is much shorter when pregnancy is terminated by spontaneous abortion. Because of this, the distribution of g must be considered as the weighted mean of two distributions: one for conceptions that do not terminate in live births and one for those that do terminate in live births. Let K_a and K_v, respectively, be the probabilities K in the two cases. Then:

$$K(\zeta,g) = [1-v(\zeta)]K_a(\zeta,g) + v(\zeta)K_v(\zeta,g). \tag{17}$$

Therefore:

$$V(x) = \pi(x)\left[1 - \int_0^G V(x-g)K_v(x-g,g)dg \right]$$

$$- \pi(x) \int_0^G V(x-g)\frac{1-v(x-g)}{v(x-g)} K_a(x-g,g)dg. \tag{18}$$

Let us consider two groups with identical effective fecundability $\pi(x)$ and probabilities K_a and K_v, but differing in the proportion of conceptions terminating in live births; let V_1, v_1, V_2 and v_2 be the functions V and v for each of these groups.

By Eq. (18), we have:

$$V_1(x)-V_2(x) = -\pi(x) \int_0^G (V_1-V_2)K_v dg$$

$$-\pi(x) \int_0^G \left(V_1\frac{1-v_1}{v_1} - V_2\frac{1-v_2}{v_2} \right)K_a dg. \tag{19}$$

Assume that v_1 is always greater than v_2. If we have:

$$V_1(x-g) < V_2(x-g),\ 0 < g \leqq G, \tag{20}$$

we then definitely have:

$$\frac{V_1(x-g)[1-v_1(x-g)]}{v_1(x-g)} < \frac{V_2(x-g)[1-v_2(x-g)]}{v_2(x-g)} \tag{21}$$

and necessarily, from Eq. (19):

$$V_1(x) > V_2(x). \tag{22}$$

If, on the contrary, we had

$$V_1(x-g) < V_2(x-g),\ 0 < g \leqq G, \tag{23}$$

we could still have

$$V_1(x) > V_2(x). \tag{24}$$

In other words, if two groups have the same effective fecundability, the one with the higher proportion of conceptions ending in live births could have an effective fertility always greater than that of the other group, but could not have a constantly lower effective fertility.

Let us now consider a central effective fertility rate analogous to the central fertility discussed in the previous section. In the simplest case, where the various fundamental functions are constant, the central effective fertility is, for a given value of effective fecundability, an increasing function of v. This central effective fertility is then equal to the reference effective fertility, i.e.

$$\frac{\pi}{1 + \bar{g}p} = \frac{\pi}{1 + \bar{g}\frac{\pi}{v}}. \tag{25}$$

$\bar{g}$ itself is a function of v. Since $\bar{g}_a$ and $\bar{g}_v$ are the mean values respectively of K_a and K_v we have

$$\bar{g} = (1-v)\bar{g}_a + v\bar{g}_v. \tag{26}$$

Thus, we finally have, for the central effective fertility:

$$\frac{\pi}{1 + \pi\bar{g}_v + \pi \frac{1-v}{v}\bar{g}_a}, \tag{27}$$

which is an expression whose value increases with v.

Now, let us consider the case where the fundamental functions vary with age. Equation (18) may be expressed in another form:

$$V(x)\left[1 + \pi(x)\int_0^G \frac{1-v}{v}K_a dg\right] = \pi(x)\left[1 - \int_0^G VK_v dg\right]$$

$$+ \pi(x)\int_0^G \Delta V \frac{1-v}{v}K_a dg \tag{28}$$

where

$$\int_0^G VK_v dg = \int_0^G V(x-g)K_v(x-g)dg$$

and

$$\Delta V = V(x)-V(x-g).$$

If the integral on the extreme right hand side of Eq. (28) containing ΔV is constantly very small, Eq. (18) would be equivalent to:

$$V(x) = \psi(x) \left[1 - \int_0^G VK_v dg \right] \qquad (29)$$

where

$$\psi(x) = \frac{\pi(x)}{1 + \pi(x) \int_0^G \frac{1-v}{v} K_a dg} .$$

Equation (29) has exactly the same form as Eq. (1), but fecundability $p(x)$ is replaced, not by the effective fecundability $\pi(x)$, but by the smaller quantity $\psi(x)$.

Under certain initial conditions, it is in fact impossible for ΔV to be sufficiently small for the solutions of Eq. (29) to become practically equal (for all x) to the solutions of Eq. (18) with the same initial conditions. Thus, in the absence of premarital conceptions, the value of $V(x)$ for x infinitely close to but greater than x_0, is equal to $\pi(x)$ in Eq. (18) and to $\psi(x)$ in Eq. (29).

On the other hand, the central solutions of Eqs. (18) and (29) can be practically identical. Let V_1 be a solution of Eq. (18) and V_2 a solution of Eq. (29) and let $D(x)$ be the difference $V_1(x) - V_2(x)$. We then have:

$$D(x) = -\psi(x) \int_0^G DK_v dg + \psi(x) \int_0^G \Delta V_1 \frac{1-v}{v} K_a dg \qquad (30)$$

which may be written as:

$$D(x) + \psi(x)\bar{g}_v\bar{D} = \psi(x) \int_0^G \Delta V_1 \frac{1-v}{v} K_a dg \qquad (31)$$

where $\bar{D}$ is the weighted average of D in the interval $(x-G,x)$ with weights $\dfrac{K_v(x-g)}{\bar{g}_v}$. [If $D(x)$ and $\bar{D}$ have the same sign, the absolute value of $D(x)$ is less than the absolute value of the right hand side of Eq. (31)—L.H.], i.e.:

$$|D(x)| < \left| \psi(x) \int_0^G \Delta V_1 \frac{1-v}{v} K_a dg \right| . \qquad (32)$$

If $D(x-g)$ is negative for $0 < g \leq G$, $D(x)$ cannot be negative if the integral in ΔV_1 is positive. In other words, when V_1 is increasing, it cannot be less than V_2 for a period longer than G; when V_1 is decreasing, it cannot be greater than V_2 for a period longer than G. In the case already mentioned where the central solutions increase, pass through a single maximum, and then decrease, V_1 will at first be above V_2 and will subsequently pass below it. Up to the point of intersection X' and starting from $X'+G$, D and $\bar{D}$ have the same sign; [we therefore know an upper limit to $D(x)$ in Eq. (32)—L.H.]. This limit is not very high since the interval where K_a is not negligible is short (conceptions not terminating in live births generally produce a relatively short nonsusceptible period). With the values used in the numerical examples, the term in ΔV is in fact negligible: for instance, it remains below [1.4 percent—L.H.] of the central effective fertility for $v = 0.8$. Equations (18) and (29) may therefore be considered as equivalent in practice, for the central solutions, but this practical equivalence does not extend to the whole set of solutions.

Before proceeding with this investigation, we believed that we could safely avoid separate consideration of the probability of conception and the frequency of spontaneous abortions and stillbirths. We believed it would suffice to use a combination of the two, i.e. the probability of a conception terminating in a live birth, together with the distribution of the duration of non-susceptibility following conceptions leading to live births (Henry [4], p. 153). It now appears that we must reckon with three fundamental functions that have distinct roles. Reducing the number of fundamental functions to two alone is justified only if, disregarding oscillations, we are interested solely in central fertilities. The fundamental function which then replaces the other two [is $\psi(x)$ as defined in Eq. (29)—L.H.] and not, as we had thought, $\pi(x)$, the probability of a conception that terminates in a live birth.

CUMULATIVE CONCEPTIONS— CUMULATIVE FERTILITY

In the absence of premarital conceptions, the mean number of conceptions by age x for a woman married at age x_0 is equal to:

$$Q(x) = \int_{x_0}^{x} C(\xi)d\xi. \tag{33}$$

The mean number of conceptions that will terminate in live births is equal to:

$$\int_{x_0}^{x} v(\xi)C(\xi)d\xi. \tag{34}$$

The average number of live births from x_0 to x, or cumulative fertility $E(x)$ by age x, is zero for $x < g_0$ and equal to:

$$E(x) = \int_{x_0}^{x-g_0} v(\xi)C(\xi)d\xi \qquad x \geqq g_0. \tag{35}$$

We have seen that the function C is the sum of the central fertility rate and a damped oscillatory function. In the absence of premarital conceptions, C is zero in the interval (x_0-G,x_0); it is below the central fertility if the latter is positive from x_0-G to x_0, which is the case for $x_0 > a+G$. Hence, at marriage, C is greater than the central fertility; the first loop of $Z(x)$, to the right of x_0, is therefore above the x-axis. $Q(x)$ is equal to the sum of the integral of the central fertility and the integral of $Z(x)$. Since the latter is a damped oscillatory function which starts with a positive loop, for $x_0 \geqq a+G$, the integral:

$$\int_{x_0}^{x} Z(\xi)d\xi$$

remains constantly positive.

For any age at marriage equal to or greater than $a+G$, the curve of cumulative conceptions remains above the curve representing the integral of the central fertility starting with marriage. This may still be the case for ages at marriage below $a+G$, but is not necessarily so.

The preceding result has an immediate application to the measurement of the phenomena; it shows that a mean pregnancy rate obtained by dividing the cumulative number of conceptions by the duration of the marriage (or by the duration of exposure to risk) is a poor index, in the sense that it may lead to erroneous interpretation. To understand this properly, let us take the particular case where neither fecundability nor the duration of nonsusceptibility varies with age. The first condition is approximately true between age x_0 and age γ, if $x_0 \geqq \beta$.

Integrating the two parts of Eq. (1) from x_0 to x, we obtain:

$$Q(x) = p \times (x-x_0) - p \int_{x_0}^{x} d\xi \int_{0}^{G} C(\xi-g)K(g)dg. \tag{36}$$

The double integral may also be written as:

$$\int_{0}^{G} K(g)dg \int_{x_0}^{x} C(\xi-g)d\xi = \int_{0}^{G} K(g)[Q(x-g)-Q(x_0-g)]dg. \tag{37}$$

Since we assume that there are no premarital conceptions, $Q(x_0-g)$ is zero and therefore we finally have:

$$Q(x) = p \times (x-x_0) - p \int_{0}^{G} Q(x-g)K(g)dg. \tag{38}$$

The function $Q(x)$ is the solution of an integral equation which differs from Eq. (1) only by the substitution of the term $p \times (x-x_0)$ for the term p. The difference between two solutions of Eq. (38) gives the same integral equation as the difference between two solutions of Eq. (1).

Equation (38) has a solution of the form $a+b \times (x-x_0)$, and by writing:[7]

$$a+b \times (x-x_0) = p \times (x-x_0) - p \int_{0}^{G} [a+b \times (x-x_0-g)]K(g)dg \tag{39}$$

it follows that:

$$a = -pa \int_{0}^{G} K(g)dg + pb \int_{0}^{G} gK(g)dg \tag{40}$$

---

[7] [The relation between these results and those in Chapter One, p. 8 (where are possibility of pregnancy wastage is ignored) may be seen as follows. Eq. (38) has a solution

$$Q(x) = a + b \times (x-x_0).$$

If all conceptions led to live births, the expected number of births by time x would be

$$E(x) = Q(x-g_0) = a+b \times (x-g_0-x_0) = a-bg_0 + b \times (x-x_0),$$

an expression with an intercept equal to $a-bg_0$, and a slope equal to ϕ' in Chapter One (see Eq. (44) below). In Chapter One, however, $E(x)$ is the expected number of births by time x after the time of marriage translated to the left by a time $g-g_0$. Therefore the intercept E_0 is equal (in terms of the notation used here) to:

$$E_0 = a-bg_0-b \times (g-g_0) = a-bg.]$$

$$b = p-pb \int_0^G K(g)dg. \tag{41}$$

The integral $\int_0^G K(g)dg$ is equal to the mean duration $\bar{g}$ of non-susceptibility, and the integral $\int_0^G gK(g)dg$ is:

$$\left[\frac{g^2}{2} K(g) \right]_0^G + \int_0^G \frac{g^2}{2} h(g)dg = \frac{\bar{g}^2 + \sigma_g^2}{2} \tag{42}$$

where σ_g^2 is the variance of g.

We finally have:[8]

$$a = b^2 \frac{\bar{g}^2 + \sigma_g^2}{2} \tag{43}$$

$$b = \frac{p}{1+\bar{g}p}. \tag{44}$$

The general solution of Eq. (38) therefore takes the form:

$$Q(x) = a+b \times (x-x_o) + \zeta(x-x_o) \tag{45}$$

where $\zeta(x-x_o)$ is a damped oscillatory function. If we divide Eq. (45) by $x-x_o$, we obtain an expression of the form:

$$\frac{Q(x)}{x-x_o} = \frac{a}{x-x_o} + b + \frac{\zeta(x-x_o)}{x-x_o} \tag{46}$$

where b is simply the central fertility, which is identical with the reference fertility in this case where the fundamental functions

---

[8] In the discrete case we have:

$$Q_x = p \left[x-x_o - \sum_{g=1}^{g=G} Q_{x-g} K_g \right]$$

giving

$$a = \frac{pb \ \Sigma \ gK_g}{1 + \bar{g}p} = \frac{pb \ [g(g+1) + \sigma_g^2]}{2 \ (1+\bar{g}p)}$$

$$b = \frac{p}{1 + \bar{g}p}$$

since

$$\Sigma gK_g = \Sigma \frac{g(g+1)}{2} h(g) = \frac{\bar{g}(\bar{g}+1)}{2} + \frac{\sigma_g^2}{2}.$$

do not vary. This is the quantity which we implicitly desired to obtain by these operations. In reality, there exists, in addition to an only slightly inconvenient oscillatory term, the hyperbolic term $a/(x-x_0)$. Thus the value of the index in Eq. (46) decreases (disregarding oscillations) as age or marital duration increases. If we are not careful at this point, we will be tempted to conclude that the same is true of the aptitude for procreation. However, in the example selected, the aptitude for procreation is assumed to be constant.

We run the same risk if, as has been recommended by some authors, we calculate legitimate fertility rates by age groups, on the basis of conceptions terminating in live births and not on the basis of live births. Thus in the case where the fundamental functions do not vary, a fertility rate might be calculated as $\dfrac{vQ(x)}{x-x_0}$. For this index, as well as that in Eq. (46), even if v is a function of x, the parasitic hyperbolic term tends to increase the fertility of those age groups in which many marriages occur, to the detriment of subsequent age groups, even if the aptitude for procreation does not appreciably vary from one to the other; hence the comparison of the two age groups 20–24 and 25–29 may be seriously distorted.

On the other hand, this risk can be greatly reduced if we work on the basis of live births. Let us return to the preceding example, and assume, moreover, that v is constant; we then have:

$$E(x) = vQ(x-g_0) = av - bvg_0 + bv \times (x-x_0) + \zeta(x-x_0-g_0). \quad (47)$$

On dividing by the duration of marriage, $x-x_0$, we obtain, disregarding the oscillatory factor, the effective central fertility bv (equivalent to the effective reference fertility in this case) if $a-bg_0$ is negligible. This condition seems to have been very nearly met in the case of the historical European populations.[9]

However, we should not believe that we can avoid all pitfalls by using live births instead of conceptions. In reality each method has its own pitfalls. For example, the calculation of fertility by year of age, on the basis of live births, may give the illusion of a maximum aptitude for procreation at a given age, even when the fundamental factors do not depend on age. One example will suffice to show this.

---

[9] [Numerical values based on observed data and used here (see Figure 6) yield $a = 0.387$, $b = 0.04$, and with $g_0 = 9$, we have $a - bg_0 = 0.027$.]

TABLE 1

POSTULATED DISTRIBUTION OF 975 MARRIAGES
PER 1,000 WOMEN, BY QUARTER AND YEAR

Quarter	Year					
	1	2	3	4	5	6
I	10	80	90	50	10	0
II	30	90	80	40	0	0
III	50	100	70	30	0	0
IV	65	100	60	20	0	0

Assume that marriages occur only when fecundability is at its plateau (at 0.2) Assume further that 90 percent of conceptions end in live births and that the duration of nonsusceptibility has the distribution given in Table 4. Let us designate the first year of age when women marry by 1, the following year by 2, etc., and let us assume that the distribution of marriages per quarter is as given in Table 1. For simplicity, suppose marriages occur at the beginning of the first month of each quarter; we obtain the expected fertility rates per woman-year shown in Table 2.

TABLE 2

ANNUAL NUMBER OF LEGITIMATE LIVE BIRTHS
PER WOMAN-YEAR OF EXPOSURE

Year	1	2	3	4	5	6	7
Fertility rate*	0.061	0.400	0.494	0.443	0.447	0.425	0.432

* Obtained by dividing the number of live births during the year by the number of woman-years; the number of woman-years is 1.0 for women married before the year in question or during the first quarter of that year, 0.75 for those married during the second quarter of the same year, 0.50 for those married during the third quarter, and 0.25 for those married during the fourth quarter.

Fertility has an apparent maximum during year 3, but since the calculations were based on the assumption that the fundamental factors are invariant, this apparent maximum has no significance with respect to the aptitude for reproduction.

NUMERICAL EXAMPLES

These examples have been treated in the discrete case, a month being taken as the time unit. The numerical values selected are

TABLE 3
POSTULATED LEVEL OF FECUNDABILITY (p) BY AGE*

Month	p	Month	p	Month	p
1	.001	25	.088	49	.178
2	.002	26	.092	50	.180
3	.004	27	.096	51	.182
4	.006	28	.100	52	.184
5	.009	29	.104	53	.186
6	.012	30	.108	54	.188
7	.016	31	.112	55	.190
8	.020	32	.116	56	.192
9	.024	33	.120	57	.194
10	.028	34	.124	58	.195
11	.032	35	.128	59	.196
12	.036	36	.132	60	.197
13	.040	37	.136	61	.198
14	.044	38	.140	62	.1985
15	.048	39	.144	63	.199
16	.052	40	.148	64	.1995
17	.056	41	.152	65	.200
18	.060	42	.156	66	.200
19	.064	43	.160	67	.200
20	.068	44	.164	68	.200
21	.072	45	.167	69	.200
22	.076	46	.170	70	.200
23	.080	47	.173	71	.200
24	.084	48	.176	72	.200

* This table refers only to the ascending section and the beginning of the plateau; age α has been labelled month number 1 and age β is month number 65; the descending section is obtained by symmetry.

of the order of magnitude of those actually encountered, or at least are plausible values.

For fecundability, a symmetrical curve was assumed (Table 3): $\alpha\beta$ and $\gamma\omega$ have the same duration; between ages β and γ, fecundability is at a plateau with a value of 20 percent, which is of the order of magnitude of the mean fecundability of newly married women aged 20–29 years. The proportion of conceptions terminating in live births was put at 90 percent; the mean value of g at 20 months in order to have a round number for the total fertility rate at the plateau (0.04 per month and 0.48 per year),[10]

---

[10] [The total fertility rate per month is $1/i$, where i, the mean interval between conceptions, is equal to $\bar{g} + \dfrac{1}{p} = 25$ when $\bar{g} = 20$ and $p = 0.20$.]

and to have for the effective fertility, a value close to observed
legitimate fertility rates of fecund women aged 20–29 years, in
historical European populations (0.40–0.45 per year).

The most difficult task was to establish the distribution of the
nonsusceptible periods. We started from the notion that the
overall distribution should be the sum of three elementary distributions corresponding to the following cases:

1. conception does not terminate in live birth.
2. a liveborn infant dies before the age of one year.
3. the infant survives its first birthday.

For each case, we constructed a rather arbitrary distribution
and subsequently modified the distributions slightly so as to obtain an overall mean of 20 months. Clearly, this result makes no
claim to accuracy. It can, however, be considered that the distribution gives an idea of what the actual distributions in the
old European populations might have been.[11] The distribution is
shown in Table 4.

The calculations were carried out only for the case where the
distribution of nonsusceptibility does not vary with age. Two
ages at marriage were considered: age α and an age when fecundability has reached its plateau, in practice, age β. In both cases, we
calculated the number of conceptions per month during the first
years of marriage. The calculations were not carried to age ω; we
assumed that the plateau lasted sufficiently long so that oscillations would practically have disappeared before age γ. Under
these conditions, conceptions in the descending section, between
age γ and ω, are the same for all ages at marriage sufficiently
below γ. They are calculated by taking 0.04 as the total fertility
rate in the last 32 months of the plateau (since G equals 32 in
Table 4).

For ages α to β, we evaluated the central fertility; the results
were obtained by trial and error and not by solving a system
of 32 equations with 32 unknowns; as a result, there are small
residual oscillations.

Figure 3 shows, in curve a, for women married at age α, the
expected monthly conceptions $C(x)$. These are compared with
the central fertility rate (curve b) and the reference fertility

---

[11] In this distribution, we assume that the 10 percent of conceptions that
fail to end in a live birth all terminate in spontaneous abortion after a
rather short pregnancy; stillbirths have been ignored, but we have assumed
an infant mortality rate of 22.2 percent (20 percent of the conceptions), including a high proportion of deaths in the first month.

TABLE 4

POSTULATED DISTRIBUTION (PER 100 PREGNANCIES)
OF THE DURATION OF NONSUSCEPTIBILITY FOR THE
THREE PREGNANCY OUTCOMES

Duration of Nonsusceptibility (fetal death)	Frequency	Duration of Nonsusceptibility (infant death)	Frequency	Duration of Nonsusceptibility (surviving live birth)	Frequency
				19 months	2
				20 months	3
				21 months	5
				22 months	7
		9 months	3	23 months	8
		10 months	6	24 months	9
		11 months	4	25 months	9
2 months	1	12 months	1	26 months	8
3 months	4	13 months	1	27 months	7
4 months	4	14 months	1	28 months	5
5 months	1	15 months	1	29 months	3
6 months	—	16 months	1	30 months	2
7 months	—	17 months	1	31 months	1
8 months	—	18 months	1	32 months	1
Total	10	Total	20	Total	70

Grand Total: 100

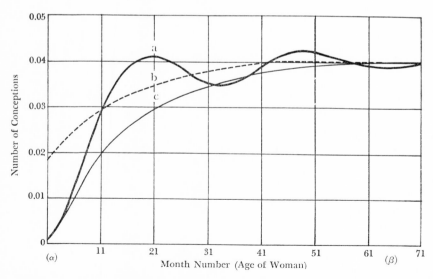

Figure 3. Expected number of conceptions per month per woman married at age α (curve a), central fertility (curve b) and reference fertility (curve c).

TABLE 5

MONTHLY NUMBER OF CONCEPTIONS PER 10,000
WOMEN MARRIED AT AGE a*

Month	Calculated No. of Conceptions	Central Fertility	Reference Fertility	Month	Calculated No. of Conceptions	Central Fertility	Reference Fertility
1.	10	184	10	37.	357	390	366
2.	20	199	19	38.	363	392	369
3.	40	211	37	39.	370	394	372
4.	60	223	54	40.	378	395	374
5.	89	234	76	41.	386	397	377
6.	117	246	97	42.	394	399	379
7.	155	258	121	43.	402	401	381
8.	190	268	143	44.	409	402	383
9.	224	276	162	45.	413	401	385
10.	256	285	179	46.	416	401	386
11.	284	293	195	47.	419	401	388
12.	310	299	209	48.	422	402	389
13.	333	306	222	49.	421	400	390
14.	353	313	234	50.	420	399	391
15.	370	319	245	51.	419	399	392
16.	384	324	255	52.	417	399	393
17.	395	329	264	53.	415	399	394
18.	402	334	273	54.	413	400	395
19.	407	339	281	55.	410	400	396
20.	410	344	288	56.	407	401	396
21.	411	348	295	57.	404	402	397
22.	408	352	302	58.	400	401	397
23.	405	356	308	59.	397	401	398
24.	400	359	314	60.	394	401	398
25.	393	363	319	61.	391	401	399
26.	386	366	324	62.	389	400	399
27.	378	369	329	63.	388	400	399
28.	370	372	333	64.	388	400	400
29.	363	374	337	65.	388	400	400
30.	357	376	341	66.	388	399	400
31.	352	378	345	67.	390	399	400
32.	348	381	349	68.	391	399	400
33.	347	383	353	69.	393	399	400
34.	347	385	356	70.	395	399	400
35.	349	387	360	71.	397	400	400
36.	352	388	363	72.	399	400	400

* Age α is equal to month number 1.

(curve c). Detailed numerical results for the three curves are given in Table 5.

Figure 3 clearly shows the oscillations of the fertility rate around central fertility, and that central fertility is greater than reference fertility. Note that central fertility is not very low when reference fertility is low; at about age α, central fertility

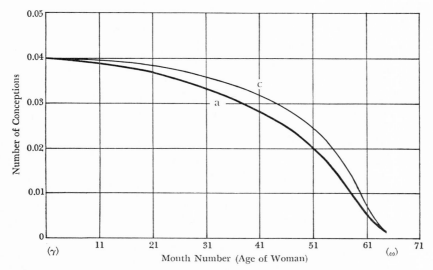

Figure 4. Expected number of conceptions per month per woman after age γ (curve a), and reference fertility (curve c).

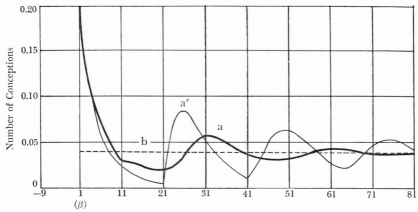

Figure 5. Expected monthly number of conceptions per month per woman married at age β (curves a and a') and central fertility (curve b). Curve a corresponds to the distribution of the duration of nonsusceptibility in Table 4; curve a' has a constant duration of nonsusceptibility equal to 20 months.

does not express "aptitude for procreation."

Figure 4 shows $C(x)$ and the reference fertility after age γ. $C(x)$ drops uniformly; as predicted, it is constantly below reference fertility. The calculations are presented in Table 6.

TABLE 6

MONTHLY NUMBER OF CONCEPTIONS
AFTER AGE γ PER 10,000 WOMEN

Month	Monthly Number of Conceptions	Reference Fertility	Month	Monthly Number of Conceptions	Reference Fertility
1.*	400	400	34.	321	349
2.	399	400	35.	316	345
3.	398	399	36.	312	341
4.	398	399	37.	307	337
5.	397	399	38.	302	333
6.	396	398	39.	296	329
7.	394	398	40.	291	324
8.	393	397	41.	285	319
9.	392	397	42.	277	314
10.	390	396	43.	270	308
11.	388	396	44.	263	302
12.	386	395	45.	256	295
13.	384	394	46.	248	288
14.	383	393	47.	240	281
15.	381	392	48.	231	273
16.	380	391	49.	222	264
17.	379	390	50.	212	255
18.	377	389	51.	201	245
19.	375	388	52.	190	234
20.	372	386	53.	178	222
21.	370	385	54.	165	209
22.	367	383	55.	152	195
23.	363	381	56.	137	179
24.	359	379	57.	122	162
25.	355	377	58.	105	143
26.	351	374	59.	87	121
27.	348	372	60.	67	97
28.	344	369	61.	52	76
29.	341	366	62.	36	54
30.	337	363	63.	25	37
31.	333	360	64.	13	19
32.	329	356	65.†	7	10
33.	325	353			

* Month number 1 coincides with age γ, when fecundability begins to decline.
† Month number 65 coincides with age ω, beyond which fecundability is zero.

Figure 5 shows the expected monthly conceptions $C(x)$ for women married at the beginning of the plateau, i.e. at age β. The data in curve a are presented in Table 7. The oscillations are very appreciable during the first four years; at the end of six or seven years of marriage, their amplitude is still about 7 percent of the central value.

TABLE 7

MONTHLY NUMBER OF CONCEPTIONS
PER 10,000 WOMEN MARRIED AT AGE β

Month	Concep-tions	Month	Concep-tions	Month	Concep-tions	Month	Concep-tions
1.*	2,000	22.	198	43.	363	64.	444
2.	1,600	23.	214	44.	351	65.	438
3.	1,280	24.	246	45.	341	66.	431
4.	1,028	25.	291	46.	333	67.	425
5.	842	26.	346	47.	327	68.	418
6.	705	27.	407	48.	324	69.	411
7.	593	28.	466	49.	323	70.	404
8.	498	29.	517	50.	326	71.	397
9.	417	30.	554	51.	333	72.	391
10.	349	31.	574	52.	343	73.	385
11.	304	32.	578	53.	355	74.	381
12.	288	33.	569	54.	369	75.	377
13.	283	34.	553	55.	385	76.	375
14.	272	35.	530	56.	402	77.	374
15.	259	36.	503	57.	416	78.	373
16.	246	37.	476	58.	428	79.	375
17.	233	38.	451	59.	438	80.	378
18.	221	39.	429	60.	445	81.	381
19.	210	40.	409	61.	449	82.	385
20.	200	41.	392	62.	449	83.	389
21.	196	42.	377	63.	448	84.	394

* Month number 1 is the first month of marriage.

Figure 5 also shows the curve a' of $C(x)$ that would be obtained if the duration of nonsusceptibility had a single value (the mean of the distribution in Table 4, i.e. 20 months) instead of stretching over the range 2 to 32 months. The oscillations around the central value 0.04, which is common to both cases, are much more pronounced in this case.

Figure 6 shows the curves of cumulative conceptions $Q(n)$ and births $E(n)$. $Q(n)$ is obtained by cumulating the conceptions in Table 7. The cumulative number of births $E(n)$ is obtained by multiplying the conceptions of month $(n-9)$ by 0.9. The value of $Q(n)$ oscillates around the central straight line, (i.e. Eq. (45) without the oscillatory part), the intercept of which (a of Eq. 45) is at 0.387. This straight line intersects the abscissa at a negative value, i.e. at $x = -9.67$. Since this value is of the order of nine months, the central straight line for the cumulative births $E(n)$ passes extremely close to the origin.

Figure 7 shows the corresponding values after dividing by n. The numerical results are given in Table 8. These results con-

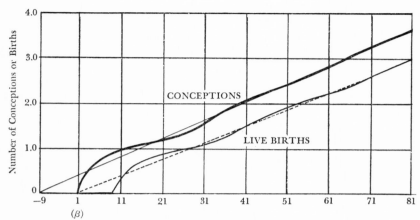

Month of Marriage (Age of Woman According to Marriage Duration in Months)

Figure 6. Cumulative number of conceptions and live births expected per woman married at age β, and the corresponding central regression lines.

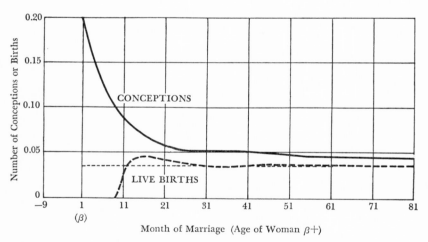

Month of Marriage (Age of Woman $\beta+$)

Figure 7. Mean number of conceptions and mean number of live births during the first n months of marriage. The horizontal asymptotes (solid and broken) represent the limits of these mean numbers for very large n.

form to theory, but this numerical example shows clearly:

(a) that the oscillations of these indices are minor after the duration of marriage exceeds two years. Also, for conceptions the oscillations are so inapparent as to be overlooked by an inexperienced observer. This pitfall is well hidden. The circum-

TABLE 8

EXPECTED CUMULATIVE CONCEPTIONS AND BIRTHS PER MONTH OF
MARRIED LIFE FOR 10,000 WOMEN MARRIED AT AGE β*

n	Conceptions	Births	n	Conceptions	Births	n	Conceptions	Births
1.	2,000	0	29.	507	367	57.	462	365
2.	1,800	0	30.	509	361	58.	462	364
3.	1,627	0	31.	511	355	59.	462	362
4.	1,477	0	32.	513	350	60.	461	361
5.	1,350	0	33.	514	346	61.	461	361
6.	1,242	0	34.	516	343	62.	461	360
7.	1,149	0	35.	516	342	63.	461	359
8.	1,068	0	36.	515	343	64.	460	359
9.	996	0	37.	514	345	65.	460	359
10.	931	180	38.	513	348	66.	459	359
11.	874	295	39.	511	352	67.	459	360
12.	825	366	40.	508	356	68.	458	360
13.	783	409	41.	505	360	69.	458	361
14.	747	434	42.	502	364	70.	457	362
15.	714	448	43.	499	367	71.	457	362
16.	685	453	44.	496	369	72.	456	363
17.	658	453	45.	492	371	73.	455	363
18.	634	448	46.	488	372	74.	454	364
19.	612	441	47.	485	373	75.	453	364
20.	591	433	48.	482	373	76.	452	364
21.	573	425	49.	479	373	77.	451	364
22.	556	417	50.	475	373	78.	450	364
23.	541	409	51.	472	372	79.	449	364
24.	528	402	52.	470	371	80.	448	364
25.	519	394	53.	468	370	81.	447	364
26.	512	387	54.	466	369	82.	446	364
27.	508	380	55.	464	368	83.	445	364
28.	506	373	56.	463	366	84.	445	363

* n designates the month number. The mean cumulative number of conceptions
or births is obtained by dividing n into the cumulative conceptions up to month n.

stances combine to tempt one to conclude from this index that
the aptitude for procreation decreases with the duration of marriage.

(b) that, even after a long duration of marriage, the mean
number of conceptions stays clearly higher (11 percent at the
end of seven years) than the central value, which characterizes
the aptitude for procreation and which is invariant by assumption.

(c) the mean number of births, on the contrary, is close to
its central value; the difference, which is about 5 percent after
three years of marriage, is only 1 percent after seven years of
marriage.

SUMMARY AND CONCLUSION

After indicating the basis for mathematical models of fertility and of family building, we investigated the fertility, in the absence of birth control, of a homogeneous group of women characterized by three functions of the woman's age (x): $p(x) =$ fecundability, $v(x) =$ the proportion of conceptions terminating in live births, and $K(x,g) =$ the probability that a woman who conceived at age x is still nonsusceptible at age $x+g$.

The main points brought out by this investigation are:

1. Two similar groups of women, married at different ages, do not have identical fertility at each age. However, the difference in the fertility of the two groups is of a special type: it is a damped oscillatory function. Hence, fertility at a given age is practically independent of age at marriage for women married at different ages if the duration of marriage is sufficiently long for all the women.

2. At very early ages, the duration of marriage cannot be long; therefore, in the analysis of fertility at such ages, we must not disregard age at marriage.

3. For women married at a given age, we can define a central solution, i.e., the solution with the least oscillations, of the fundamental integral equation. Legitimate fertility after this age is then the sum of this central solution and of a damped oscillatory function. After a very long marital duration, the central solution and the actual fertility practically coincide.

The central solution defined for women married at a given age x_0 is not necessarily identical, after x_0, with the central solution for women married at another age less than x_0; the difference is a damped oscillatory function.

There is an advantage in selecting a unique central solution, obviously the one corresponding to the lowest age at marriage, when fecundability ceases to be zero. This solution has been called central fertility.

4. Central fertility, as defined here, is a mathematical entity. It would be surprising if observed fertility were identical with central fertility at short marital durations. Especially at very early ages, central fertility may not be zero, whereas fecundability is infinitely small.

5. On the assumption that central fertility is known, it fur-

nishes little information on the development, with age, of the aptitude for procreation. This reason alone (there are others) would be sufficient to justify great caution in interpreting apparently smooth curves of fertility by age, in terms of aptitude.

6. In the absence of premarital conceptions, the expected cumulative number of conceptions at the end of t years of marriage (t very large) is greater than the integral from zero to t of the central fertility for all women married after age $a+G$, in which a is the age when fecundability ceases to be zero.

In the case, particularly interesting with respect to the historical European populations, where marriage occurs during the age period when fecundability is at a plateau, the mean number of conceptions per unit of time during the first x years of marriage (obtained by dividing x into the cumulative number of conceptions up to time x) is a decreasing function of x, disregarding oscillations. In other words, certain indices of fertility using conceptions may decrease with increasing marital duration, even though the aptitude for procreation is constant. For this reason, an index of fertility using live births is preferable; the misleading decrease does not occur. However, if indices for shorter intervals, such as one year, are calculated, there is a risk of obtaining a maximum value, which is due solely to the combination of fertility oscillations and the distribution of marriages by age. It has no significance regarding the aptitude for procreation.

In summary, mathematical models show primarily that results from a study of legitimate fertility must be interpreted with great caution, since the relations between legitimate fertility and those fundamental functions that define the aptitude for procreation are complex. Special care is needed in the study of fertility at very young ages, below age 20 and even between 20–24 years of age, if most marriages occur in this age group rather than in the earlier one. Because of unavoidable oscillations in fertility at the beginning of marriage, rates calculated for short intervals, such as one year, rather than rates for five-year age groups, are not necessarily an improvement. Since five-year rates themselves are only a very rough index for women under age 20, it would seem once more that investigation of fertility at these ages requires special methods.

At ages when fecundability is at a plateau or does not change quickly, five-year rates eliminate or attenuate the oscillations without distorting the curve of fertility by age; they are preferable to rates by year of age. Finally, it is only when fecundability is decreasing, and particularly after age 40, that short period rates may be preferable to five-year rates. At these ages, for nearly all women, the duration of marriage is sufficiently long that the influence of the early oscillations is no longer felt.

CHAPTER THREE

Fertility and Family:

Mathematical Models II*

EDITORS' SUMMARY

This chapter (published in 1961) amalgamates, in translation, a paper that was originally published in two parts. It is directed in particular to an investigation of: (a) the distribution of cumulative fertility, according to the duration of marriage, (b) the mean intervals between births that occur in an age period (or marital duration) of finite length, (c) the mean lengths of intervals that "straddle" an age period, (d) the relation between completed parity and interval length, and (e) the effect of a period of declining fecundability, toward the end of reproductive life, on the mean lengths of the intervals between the last several births. The models are illustrated by numerical calculations and the results are compared with several sets of empirical data.

*Originally printed in French as "Fecondité et famille. Modèles mathématiques (II)." *Population* 16, no. 1 (Janv.-Mars 1961): 27-48, and *Population* 16, no. 2 (Avril-Juin 1961): 261-282.

CONTENTS

Theoretical Aspects

[THE ASSUMPTIONS in this chapter are the same as in Chapter Two.][1]

CONCEPTIONS AND LIVE BIRTHS BY ORDER

Let $C_k\ dx$ be the expected number of conceptions of order k in the age interval $(x, x + dx)$. $C_k\ dx$ is equal to pdx times the number of women exposed to conception for the kth time. For $k \geq 2$, the only such women are those who have conceived $k - 1$

---

[1] [The recapitulation of the assumptions in the French text has been omitted here.]

SUMMARY OF NOTATION

(all "risks" defined below refer to instantaneous occurrence rates)

x or ξ	Age.
$C(x)$	Risk of a conception at age x.
$C_k(x)$	Risk of a kth conception at age x.
$C_{nk}(x)$	Risk of a kth conception at age x for a woman whose completed parity will be equal to n.
$\mathbf{C}_{x_0}(x)$	Risk of a conception at age x given that the most recent conception occurred at age x_0.
$\mathbf{C}_t(u - t)$	Risk of a conception at time u given that the most recent conception occurred at time t.
V	Pertaining to conceptions, signifies a conception that will terminate in a live birth.
$V(x)$	Risk of a V conception at age x.
$\mathbf{V}_{x_0}(x)$	Risk of a V conception at age x given that the most recent V conception occurred at age x_0.
$p(x)$	Fecundability at age x.
$\bar{p}_h(\omega)$	Harmonic mean of $p(x)$ from time of marriage until time ω.
$v(x)$	Probability that a conception occurring at age x will terminate in a live birth.
$\mathbf{P}_{k,\,c}(x)$	Probability that a conception occurring at age x will be followed by exactly k conceptions.
$\mathbf{P}_{k,\,v}(x)$	Analogous probability relating to V conceptions.
g	Duration of the nonsusceptible period.
g_a and g_v	Duration of the nonsusceptible period in the case of an A conception (terminating in abortion) and in the case of a V conception (terminating in live birth) respectively.
$k(g)$	P.d.f. of g.
$K(\xi, x - \xi)$	Probability that a woman who conceived at age ξ is still nonsusceptible at age x.
K_a and K_v	Corresponding probability in the case of an A conception and a V conception at age x respectively.
u_g	Mean duration of conception delay.
i, x	Length of an interval between conceptions.

$h(i), h(x)$ Corresponding densities.

$R(i), H(x)$ Probability of an interval greater than (i) or (x). [For convenience, the original notation using the two symbols has been retained.]

$Q_k(x)$ Total number of conceptions of order k by time x.

$E_n(x_1)$ Total number of V conceptions of order n by time x_1.

ω Arbitrary upper age limit. It is also used to designate a period sufficiently long to study straddling and interior intervals.

v Right fraction of a straddling interval. [Note: this symbol is also used for the probability that a conception will terminate in a live birth.]

r Left fraction of a straddling interval.

j Length of interior interval.

y Length of the straddling interval.

f Fertility rate in the period ω.

n_i Number of children born in the period ω to the ith woman.

γ and γ_ω Coefficients of variation of the distribution of the intervals starting either at the beginning or after ω respectively.

Where no misunderstanding can result, we sometimes take the liberty of not specifying the variable on which the function depends; we then simply write C instead of $C(x)$ or $C(\xi)$, and K instead of $K(\xi, x - \xi)$.

In the discrete case, we utilize the same symbols except here age x acts as subscript. C_x and p_x are, for example, the number of conceptions and the probability of conception during the xth unit of time. As in the continuous case, the letter x may be omitted if there is no doubt as to the applicable variable.

times but not k times, excluding those who are still in the non-susceptible state following their $(k - 1)$th conception. If x_0 is the age at marriage, the number of women who have conceived $k - 1$ times by age x is equal to:

$$Q_{k-1}(x) = \int_{x_0}^{x} C_{k-1} \, d\xi. \tag{1}$$

The number expected to have conceived k times is:

$$Q_k(x) = \int_{x_0}^{x} C_k \, d\xi, \tag{2}$$

and the number expected to be in the nonsusceptible state following the $(k-1)$th conception is:

$$\int_{x_0}^{x} C_{k-1} K d\xi. \tag{3}$$

Therefore, for $k \geqq 2$:

$$C_k = p \int_{x_0}^{x} (C_{k-1} - C_k - C_{k-1} K) \, d\xi. \tag{4}$$

For $k = 1$, in the absence of premarital conceptions, all the women except those who have already conceived, are exposed to the risk of a first conception. If the original number is put equal to unity, we therefore have:

$$C_1 = p \left(1 - \int_{x_0}^{x} C_1 \, d\xi \right). \tag{5}$$

In the discrete case, Eq. (4) and (5) are replaced by:

$$C_k = p. \sum_{\xi = x_0}^{\xi = x - 1} (C_{k-1} - C_k - C_{k-1} K) \qquad \text{when } k \geqq 2 \tag{6}$$

and

$$C_1 = p \left(1 - \sum_{\xi = x_0}^{\xi = x - 1} C_1 \right). \tag{7}$$

We now turn to live births; their order depends only on the number of preceding live births. Consequently, live births of a given order correspond to conceptions of the same or higher orders. To avoid the minor difficulty of the interval (assumed constant), between conception and live birth, we substitute conceptions terminating in live births (which we call V conceptions) for births. Also we designate as A conceptions those that terminate in abortion or stillbirth.

The expected number of V conceptions of order k in the interval $(x, x + dx)$ is equal to $pvdx$ times the number of women who have had V conceptions $(k - 1)$ times and are susceptible to a V conception of order k between x and $x + dx$. This number of women is equal to the total number of women who have had V conceptions exactly $(k - 1)$ times, reduced by:

   (a) The number of women who cannot yet have a kth V conception because they are still in the nonsusceptible state following the $(k - 1)$th V conception, and

   (b) The number of women who cannot have a kth V conception because they have too recently had an A conception.

The total number of women who had V conceptions exactly $(k - 1)$ times between marriage and age x is equal to:

$$\int_{x_0}^{x} (V_{k-1} - V_k)\, d\xi \qquad \text{for } k \geq 2 \tag{8}$$

and to:

$$1 - \int_{x_0}^{x} V_1\, d\xi \qquad \text{for } k = 1. \tag{9}$$

The number (a) of women still in the nonsusceptible state after the $(k - 1)$th V conception is equal to:

$$\int_{x_0}^{x} V_{k-1} K_v\, d\xi \qquad \text{for } k \geq 2, \tag{10}$$

and to zero for $k = 1$.

We still need to calculate the number (b) of women who are in the category V_{k-1}, and still in the nonsusceptible state following an A conception. Among women of the category V_{k-1} who conceive at a given time, v conceive a live-born infant and leave the category V_{k-1} to enter the category V_k; $(1 - v)$ have a conception that will end in abortion and remain in the category V_{k-1}. In other words, during an interval $(x, x + dx)$, the number of women who conceive without leaving the category V_{k-1} is equal to $(1 - v)/v$ times the number of women who do leave this category. The number (b) is consequently equal to:

$$\int_{x_0}^{x} \frac{1 - v}{v} V_k K_a\, d\xi. \tag{11}$$

For $k = 1$, we accordingly have:

$$V_1 = pv \left[1 - \int_{x_0}^{x} \left(V_1 + \frac{1 - v}{v} V_1 K_a \right) d\xi \right], \tag{12}$$

and for $k \geq 2$:

$$V_k = pv \left[\int_{x_0}^{x} \left(V_{k-1} - V_k - V_{k-1} K_v - \frac{1-v}{v} V_k K_a \right) d\xi \right].$$

(13)

For the discrete case, the equivalent of the above formulas is:

$$V_1 = pv \left[1 - \sum_{x_0}^{x-1} \left(V_1 + \frac{1-v}{v} V_1 K_a \right) \right]$$

(14)

$$V_k = pv \left[\sum_{x_0}^{x-1} \left(V_{k-1} - V_k - V_{k-1} K_v - \frac{1-v}{v} V_k K_a \right) \right].$$

(15)

SUCCESSIVE CONCEPTIONS
AND LIVE BIRTHS

Instead of starting with marriage, let us start with conceptions occurring at age x_0. Let us take their number as unity and $\mathbf{C}_{x_0}$ as the expected number [density] of first conceptions following x_0 that occur in $(x, x + dx)$. [In other words, if reproduction were to continue indefinitely (i.e. to infinity) without the supervention of sterility, then $\mathbf{C}_{x_0}(x)$ would be the probability density (p.d.f.) of an interval of length $(x - x_0)$ following a conception at x_0 and $\int_{x_0}^{\infty} \mathbf{C}_{x_0}(x)\, dx = 1.$] Reasoning as above, we write in the continuous case:

$$\mathbf{C}_{x_0} = p \left[1 - K(x_0, x - x_0) - \int_{x_0}^{x} \mathbf{C}_{x_0}\, d\xi \right]$$

(16)

and, in the discrete case:

$$\mathbf{C}_{x_0} = p \left[1 - K_{x_0,\, x - x_0} - \sum_{x_0}^{x-1} \mathbf{C}_{x_0} \right].$$

(17)

We now go on to live births. Assume that a V conception occurred at x_0. Let $\mathbf{V}_{x_0}$ be the expected number of first V conceptions following x_0 that occur in $(x, x + dx)$. We then have, in the continuous case:

$$\mathbf{V}_{x_0} = pv \left[1 - K_v(x_0, x - x_0) - \int_{x_0}^{x} \left[1 + \frac{1 - v}{v} K_a(x_0, \xi - x_0) \right] \mathbf{V}_{x_0} \, d\xi \right]$$

$$(18)$$

and in the discrete case:

$$\mathbf{V}_{x_0} = pv \left[1 - K_{v, \, x_0, \, x \, - \, x_0} - \sum_{x_0}^{x - 1} \left(1 + \frac{1 - v}{v} K_{a, \, x_0, \, \xi \, - x_0} \right) \mathbf{V}_{x_0} \right].$$

$$(19)$$

INTERVALS BETWEEN CONCEPTIONS
AND BETWEEN BIRTHS

We will now be concerned with establishing the distribution of intervals between conceptions or between births in cases where reproduction does not go on indefinitely. For example, assume that we are concerned with the distribution of those intervals that end before a limiting age ω, where ω may have different definitions depending on the problem being investigated. The distribution of such intervals can be established on the basis of the quantities $\mathbf{C}_{x_0}$ and $\mathbf{V}_{x_0}$. In the continuous case, the p.d.f. is equal to $\mathbf{C}_{x_0}(x)$ or $\mathbf{V}_{x_0}(x)$ divided by the total number of conceptions or births between age x_0 and the limiting age ω.

MEAN INTERVAL

For a nonsusceptible period of duration g, the mean interval between two conceptions is equal to the sum of g plus u_g, where u_g is the mean interval from the end of the nonsusceptible period to the subsequent conception, i.e., the conception delay or the mean duration of exposure to the risk of conception beginning at $x_0 + g$. Let the number of women who leave the nonsusceptible state at $x_0 + g$ be taken as unity and let $R(x)$ be the probability of not having conceived yet between $x_0 + g$ and x. We then have.[2]

$$dR = -pR \, dx. \qquad (20)$$

---

[2] [This equality follows from the fact that $R(x + dx) = R(x) (1 - p) \, dx$]. Equation (20) makes it possible to express R as a function of p. By putting:

$$P(x) = \int_{0}^{x} p \, d\zeta,$$

we obtain:

$$R(x) = \exp. \, [-P(x) + P(x_0 + g)].$$

Since the expected number of conceptions during $(x, x + dx)$ is equal to $-dR$, the mean duration of exposure to risk, u_g, is given by the equation:

$$u_g = \frac{- \int_{x_0 + g}^{\omega} (x - x_0 - g)\, dR}{1 - R(\omega)}. \tag{21}$$

After integration by parts, the numerator of Eq. (21) becomes:

$$-(\omega - x_0 - g)\, R(\omega) + \int_{x_0 + g}^{\omega} R\, dx. \tag{22}$$

The second term of this expression, i.e. the integral, may be written as:

$$\int_{x_0 + g}^{\omega} \frac{1}{p(x)} \cdot p(x)\, R\, dx. \tag{23}$$

In this form, the integral represents the product of $1 - R(\omega)$ by the inverse of a weighted harmonic mean of $p(x)$, with weights equal to the expected conceptions during $(x, x + dx)$, that is, to $p(x)\, R(x)\, dx$. Letting $\bar{p}_h(\omega)$ be the harmonic mean in question, this becomes:

$$u_g = \frac{1}{\bar{p}_h(\omega)} - \frac{(\omega - x_0 - g)\, R(\omega)}{1 - R(\omega)}, \tag{24}$$

which is reduced to $1/\bar{p}_h(\omega)$ in the case where $R(\omega)$ is either zero or so small that $(\omega - x_0 - g)\, R(\omega)$ is negligible.[3]

---

[3] To change to the discrete case, we begin by changing the origin, by giving the number 1 to the first unit of time after the nonsusceptible period, which previously had the number $(x_0 + g + 1)$, and by letting C_t be the number of conceptions in the time unit t. We have to calculate:

$$\sum_1^u t\, C_t$$

which may also be written as

$$\sum_1^u u\, C_t - \sum_1^u (u - t)\, C_t.$$

Let us put:

$$Q_{u + 1} = \sum_1^u C_t.$$

The first sum is equal to $u\, Q_{u + 1}$. The second contains $(u - 1)C_1$, $(u - 2)C_2$, ... and is consequently equal to $Q_u + Q_{u-1} + \ldots + Q_2$; Q_1, which
(continued on next page)

If ω is sufficiently large, $\bar{p}_h(\omega)$ is practically equal to the value $\bar{p}_h$ which would be obtained given infinite time; if the term in $R(\omega)$ is at the same time small enough, u_g reduces to the value $1/\bar{p}_h$.

We can derive another expression for the mean conception delay when the conception occurs within a time ω after the end of nonsusceptibility. If $h(i)$ is the p.d.f. of the interval between events (births or conceptions), and $R(i)$ is the probability of an interval greater than i, we have, using integration by parts:

$$\int_0^\omega ih\,di = \Big[\, iR \,\Big]_\omega^0 + \int_0^\omega R\,di = \int_0^\infty R\,di - \int_\omega^\infty R\,di - \omega\,R(\omega).$$

(25)

Designate by $\bar{i}_0\omega$, $\bar{i}_0$, $\bar{i}\omega$, the mean intervals respectively between zero and ω, starting with zero, and starting with ω, i.e.,

---

is zero, may be added to this sum and we can then write

$$\overset{u}{\underset{1}{\Sigma}}\, Q_t.$$

We then have:

$$\overset{u}{\underset{1}{\Sigma}}\, tC_t = u\,Q_{u+1} - \overset{u}{\underset{1}{\Sigma}}\, Q_t.$$

Since R_t is the number of women that have not conceived before the beginning of the time unit t, we have $R_t = 1 - Q_t$ and therefore

$$\overset{u}{\underset{1}{\Sigma}}\, t\,C_t = u(1 - R_{u+1}) - \overset{u}{\underset{1}{\Sigma}}\,(1 - R_t) = \overset{u}{\underset{1}{\Sigma}}\, R_t - u\,R_{u+1}.$$

We further have:

$$C_t = p_t\,R_t.$$

This finally gives:

$$\overset{u}{\underset{1}{\Sigma}}\, t\,C_t = \overset{u}{\underset{1}{\Sigma}}\, \frac{C_t}{p_t} - u\,R_{u+1},$$

which must be divided by $\overset{u}{\underset{1}{\Sigma}}\, C_t$, which may also be written as $1 - R_{u+1}$.

We arrive at a formula analogous to the one obtained in the continuous case, [equation added in translation], i.e.,

$$u_g = \frac{\overset{u}{\underset{1}{\Sigma}}\, t\,C_t}{\overset{u}{\underset{1}{\Sigma}}\, C_t} = \frac{1}{1 - R_{u+1}}\left[\,\overset{u}{\underset{1}{\Sigma}}\, \frac{C_t}{p_t} - u\,R_{u+1}\right] = \frac{1}{\bar{p}_{h(u)}} - \frac{u\,R_{u+1}}{1 - R_{u+1}}$$

$$\bar{i}_{0\omega} = \frac{\int_0^\omega ih(i)\,di}{\int_0^\omega h(i)\,di} = \frac{\int_0^\omega R(i)\,di}{1 - R(\omega)} \tag{26}$$

$$\bar{i}_0 = \int_0^\infty ih(i)\,di = \int_0^\infty R(i)\,di, \tag{27}$$

and

$$\bar{i}_\omega = \frac{\int_\omega^\infty (i - \omega)h(i)\,di}{\int_\omega^\infty h(i)\,di} = \frac{\int_\omega^\infty R(i)\,di}{R(\omega)}, \tag{28}$$

we then have, from Eq. (25):

$$[1 - R(\omega)]\,\bar{i}_{0\omega} = \bar{i}_0 - R(\omega)\,(\omega + \bar{i}_\omega) \tag{29}$$

and therefore:

$$\bar{i}_{0\omega} = \bar{i}_0 - \frac{R(\omega)\,[\omega + \bar{i}_\omega - \bar{i}_0]}{1 - R(\omega)}. \tag{30}$$

Equation (30) is reduced to $\bar{i}_0$ when the term in $R(\omega)$ is sufficiently small. When fecundability is constant, $\bar{i}_\omega = \bar{i}_0$, and Eq. (30) is reduced to $\bar{i}_0 - \dfrac{\omega\,R(\omega)}{1 - R(\omega)}$.

The mean interval between conceptions is equal to the sum $g + u_g$, for a specific value g of the duration of nonsusceptibility. For all possible values, if h is the p.d.f. of g, this mean interval is equal to:

$$\frac{\int_0^{\omega - x_0} (g + u_g)\,h\,dg}{\int_0^{\omega - x_0} h\,dg}. \tag{31}$$

If $\omega - x_0$ is sufficiently large, this mean interval is equal to the sum of $\bar{g}(x_0)$, the mean nonsusceptible period starting at x_0, and the weighted mean of [the inverse] of the harmonic means, i.e. of $\dfrac{1}{\bar{p}_h(\omega)}$.

The mean interval between two V conceptions has a more complicated expression; we shall restrict ourselves to the following special case.

SPECIAL CASE

In this special case the fundamental functions p, K, and v are independent of x and the duration $\omega - x_0$ is sufficiently long to be treated as infinite.

The mean time to conception is $1/p$, and the mean interval between two conceptions is $\bar{g} + 1/p$. The mean interval between two conceptions terminating in live births is equal to $\bar{g}_v + 1/p$, when they are not separated by an abortion; it is equal to $\bar{g}_v + 1/p + \bar{g}_a + 1/p = \bar{g}_v + \bar{g}_a + 2/p$ when they are separated by one abortion, and to $\bar{g}_v + 1/p + n(\bar{g}_a + 1/p)$ when they are separated by n abortions, where $\bar{g}$, $\bar{g}_v$, $\bar{g}_a$ are the mean values for total conceptions, V conceptions, and A conceptions respectively. The probability of the first case is v, that of the second one is $(1 - v)\,v$, and that of the third case (n abortions) is $(1 - v)^n\,v$. From this, we derive for the value of the mean interval:

$$\bar{\imath} = v(\bar{g}_v + 1/p) + v(1 - v)\,(\bar{g}_v + \bar{g}_a + 2/p) +$$

$$\dots + v(1 - v)^n \left[\bar{g}_v + n\bar{g}_a + \frac{n + 1}{p} \right] + \dots \tag{32}$$

$$= \bar{g}_v + 1/p + \frac{(1 - v)}{v}\,(\bar{g}_a + 1/p) = (\bar{g} + 1/p)/v.$$

SEQUENCE OF THREE CONCEPTIONS OR THREE BIRTHS

[Let us suppose that three conceptions occur respectively at ages x, ξ and ζ. Taking the first conception as the origin, we assume that the three consecutive conceptions occur at the times 0, $(t, t + dt)$, $(u, u + du)$, where $t = \xi - x$ and $u = \zeta - x$.] The probability of such a sequence (given that the first conception occurred at 0) is equal to:

$$\mathbf{C}_0\,(t)\,\mathbf{C}_t\,(u - t)\,dt\,du, \tag{33}$$

where $\mathbf{C}_0$ is the density of the time interval t, between the conception at t and the original conception, and $\mathbf{C}_t$ is the density of the interval $(u - t)$ between the conception at u and the preceding conception at t.

Let us fix the value of u. The p.d.f. of the interval t becomes:

$$\frac{\mathbf{C}_0\,(t)\,\mathbf{C}_t\,(u - t)\,dt}{\displaystyle\int_0^u \mathbf{C}_0\,(t)\,\mathbf{C}_t\,(u - t)\,dt}. \tag{34}$$

We seek the mean value of t; for this purpose, we must calculate the value of the integral:

$$\int_0^u t\mathbf{C}_0(t)\,\mathbf{C}_t(u-t)\,dt. \tag{35}$$

Let us start with the case where the density of the interval $(u-t)$ is equal to the density of a t interval of equal magnitude. The integral (Eq. 35) then becomes

$$\int_0^u t\mathbf{C}_0(t)\,\mathbf{C}_0(u-t)\,dt = \int_0^u (u-t)\,\mathbf{C}_0(t)\,\mathbf{C}_0(u-t)\,dt,$$

$$\tag{36}$$

where the right hand side is the numerator for the mean of the interval that separates the second conception at t from the third conception at u. Hence, the two successive mean intervals, i.e., that between the first and second, and that between the second and third conceptions, are equal in this case and the mean of t is equal to $u/2$.

This result holds for the case where the fundamental functions are independent of age, at least in a fairly long age span, i.e., when fecundability, the distribution of duration of nonsusceptibility, and the risk of pregnancy wastage remain constant within this long age span. For a series of at least three births within this age span, the mean interval between two consecutive births is independent of the order of these births in this series. If, for example, the fundamental functions are independent of age between 20 and 35 years, the mean interval between births of order [equal to or −L.H.] less than 5 is independent of order, in families where the woman had five births between her twentieth and her thirty-fifth birthday. In other words, the mean intervals 1–2, 2–3, 3–4, 4–5 are equal in these families.

Let us now consider the case where there is a correlation between the lengths of the two intervals, in a manner such that with increasing age at the earlier conception, the distribution of the time to the next conception is increasingly shifted to the right. In that case, $\mathbf{C}_0$ is less spread out in any interval smaller than u than [$\mathbf{C}_t$ −L.H.] would be in the same interval. As a result, $\mathbf{C}_0\mathbf{C}_t$ is the product of two functions such as $\mathbf{C}_0$ and $\mathbf{C}_t$ in Figure 1.

On the right hand side of the figure, the curve $\mathbf{C}_t(u-t)$ is located below the curve [$\mathbf{C}'_0$ −L.H.] which is the mirror image of

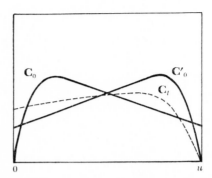

Figure 1. Schematic representation of a case where C_t is shifted to the right as compared with C_0. C'_0 *is the mirror image of* C_0.

C_0. On the left, however, C_t is above C'_0. The product $C_0 \ C_t$ is consequently an asymmetric distribution, concentrated on the left with a mean less than $u/2$.

Thus, if a series of births occur within a long age span, and if the fundamental functions change within this age span so that the spread of the distribution of conception intervals increases with age, the mean intervals between two successive births increase with birth order. This is true, for example, if fecundability constantly decreases with age in the span under consideration. The reverse would occur if the spread of the distribution diminished with age.

NUMBER OF BIRTHS IN A FAMILY

Let us consider an age $x_1 > x_0$, where x_0 is the age at marriage. Then from Eq. (1), the expected number of conceptions of order n by age x_1 is equal to:

$$Q_n (x_1) = \int_{x_0}^{x_1} C_n \, dx, \tag{1'}$$

in the continuous case, and to:

$$Q_{n, x_1} = \sum_{x_0}^{x_1 - 1} C_n, \tag{37}$$

in the discrete case. We designate it as $Q_n(x_1)$, Q_{n, x_1}, or, more simply, as Q_n.

Analogous formulas may be derived for conceptions terminating in live births. In the continuous case, the expected number of such conceptions of order n by age x_1, denoted $E_n(x_1)$, or simply E_n, is equal to:

$$E_n(x_1) = \int_{x_0}^{x_1} V_n \, dx, \qquad (38)$$

and in the discrete case, $E_{n,\,x_1}$ or E_n is equal to:

$$E_{n,\,x_1} = \sum_{x_0}^{x_1 - 1} V_n. \qquad (39)$$

Let us now consider Q_n and Q_{n+1}. $Q_n(x_1)$ is necessarily greater than $Q_{n+1}(x_1)$ because some of the women who conceived n times have not had time for the $(n+1)$th conception, especially if the nth conception has occurred very shortly before x_1. However, the difference may be small.[4]

The difference $Q_n - Q_{n+1}$ is therefore equal to the expected proportion of women who have conceived exactly n times during the duration of marriage $x_1 - x_0$. In the same way, $E_n - E_{n+1}$ is equal to the expected proportion of women who have had (with a time shift of about nine months) exactly n live births.

COMPLETED FERTILITY

Let ω be the age after which fecundability is zero; the family has then been completed. The distribution of completed fertility, by the number of conceptions or live births, is obtained by determining the successive differences:

or

$$1 - Q_1(\omega), \ Q_1(\omega) - Q_2(\omega) \dots$$
$$\qquad (40)$$
$$1 - E_1(\omega), \ E_1(\omega) - E_2(\omega) \dots$$

In practice, the number of conceptions and, *a fortiori,* of births cannot exceed a given limit; $Q_n(\omega)$ is therefore zero beyond a given value u of n, and $E_n(\omega)$ is zero beyond a value v; the last non-zero term of the first series is Q_u and that of the second is E_v.

LAST CONCEPTION AND LAST BIRTH

[Consider women who conceive at age x. If x is sufficiently near

---

[4] [If $x_1 - x_0$ is relatively long, and n is not large, then it is possible that $Q_n = Q_{n+1} = 1$. In other words, for example, if the duration of marriage is 20 years, all women may have at least two conceptions and therefore $Q_1 = Q_2 = 1$. Hence we can say only that Q_n is not less than Q_{n+1}.]

the highest fecund age, ω, a non-negligible proportion of these women will have no other conception and then $\displaystyle\sum_{\xi = x + 1}^{\xi = \omega} \mathbf{C}_{x, \xi}$ is not equal to 1. (In this expression, $\mathbf{C}_{x, \xi}$ represents the number of conceptions at age ξ per woman who had conceived at age x.)

The difference:

$$1 - \sum_{\xi = x + 1}^{\xi = \omega} \mathbf{C}_{x, \xi} = \mathbf{P}_{x, 0, c} \qquad (41)$$

is equal to the probability that a woman who conceives at age x, will not conceive again.]

Multiplying the conceptions C by $\mathbf{P}_{x, 0, c}$, we obtain the expected number of last conceptions C_u.

Similarly, we calculate the probability $\mathbf{P}_{x, 0, v}$ that a conception terminating in live birth will be the last, and, multiplying V by $\mathbf{P}_{x, 0, v}$, we calculate the last V conceptions, V_u.

Since fecundity at any time is, by hypothesis, independent of parity, the probability that a conception will not be followed by any others is independent of its order. Multiplying C_n by $\mathbf{P}_{x, 0, v}$, we obtain the last conceptions of order n, $C_{n, u}$. Similarly, the product $V_n \mathbf{P}_{x, 0, v}$ gives us, with a shift in time, the live births of order n that are the last ones, i.e. the last births in n child families.

Order of Birth and Final Size of Families

The last births in n child families are the births of order n in families of size n. However, we might be equally interested in the second last birth of order $n - 1$, and in general, in the births of each order $\leqq n$ in n-child families. Besides, we shall see from the numerical examples that it is essential to combine birth order with the final size of families if we are to avoid errors of interpretation which are both serious and frequent.

If a conception or a birth is the second last, the subsequent conception or birth is the last one. A conception following age x can occur at an age ξ equal to $x + 1$, $x + 2$, ..., $\omega - 1$ or ω; for a given value of ξ, the probability that it will be the last is $\mathbf{P}_{\xi, 0, c}$ analogous to $\mathbf{P}_{x, 0, c}$; that is,

$$\mathbf{P}_{x, 1, c} = \sum_{\xi = x + 1}^{\xi = \omega} \mathbf{P}_{\xi, 0, c} \, \mathbf{C}_{x, \xi} . \qquad (42)$$

In the continuous case, we write:

$$\mathbf{P}_{1,\,c}(x) = \int_{x}^{\omega} \mathbf{C}_{x}(\xi)\,\mathbf{P}_{0,\,c}(\xi)\,d\xi \tag{43}$$

Analogous formulas are obtained for births by replacing $\mathbf{C}_x$ by $\mathbf{V}_x$, $\mathbf{P}_{x,\,0,\,c}$ and $\mathbf{P}_{x,\,1,\,c}$ by $\mathbf{P}_{x,\,0,\,v}$ and $\mathbf{P}_{x,\,1,\,v}$ respectively.

Once $\mathbf{P}_{1,\,c}$ [omitting the subscript x] is calculated, the same procedure can be utilized to calculate $\mathbf{P}_{2,\,c}$, i.e. the probability that a conception may be followed by only two more or, in other words, that it will be the third from the last.

In general, the probability $\mathbf{P}_{k,\,c}$ that a conception will be followed by k and only k other conceptions is given by:

$$\mathbf{P}_{k,\,c} = \int_{x}^{\omega} \mathbf{C}_x\,\mathbf{P}_{k\,-\,1,\,c}\,d\xi \tag{44}$$

or

$$\mathbf{P}_{k,\,c} = \sum_{\xi\,=\,x\,+\,1}^{\xi\,=\,\omega} \mathbf{C}_x\,\mathbf{P}_{k\,-\,1,\,c}. \tag{45}$$

Similarly, we have:

$$\mathbf{P}_{k,\,v} = \int_{x}^{\omega} \mathbf{V}_x\,\mathbf{P}_{k\,-\,1,\,v}\,d\xi \tag{46}$$

$$\mathbf{P}_{k,\,v} = \sum_{x\,+\,1}^{\omega} \mathbf{V}_x\,\mathbf{P}_{k\,-\,1,\,v}. \tag{47}$$

Thus, we can obtain, on the basis of the fundamental functions and through the quantities $\mathbf{C}_x(\xi)$ and $\mathbf{V}_x(\xi)$, tables of the probabilities $\mathbf{P}_{0,\,c}$, $\mathbf{P}_{1,\,c}$, . . ., $\mathbf{P}_{k,\,c}$ and $\mathbf{P}_{0,\,v}$, $\mathbf{P}_{1,v}$, . . ., $\mathbf{P}_{k,\,v}$.

These tables can be utilized for any size or group of sizes of the family. If we need to calculate, for example, births 1 to 11 in 11-child families, we would, for each value of x, determine the products:

$$\mathbf{V}_{11}\,\mathbf{P}_{0,\,v},\ \mathbf{V}_{10}\,\mathbf{P}_{1,\,v},\ \mathbf{V}_{9}\,\mathbf{P}_{2,\,v},\,\dots\,,\,\mathbf{V}_{1}\,\mathbf{P}_{10,\,v}.$$

To calculate results for all last births, we multiple $\mathbf{V}$ by $\mathbf{P}_{0,\,v}$; but if we require also results for the second last births, we have to limit ourselves to those families in which there actually are second last births, i.e. to women that have had a least two live births.

FERTILITY RATES
AND INTERVALS BETWEEN BIRTHS

In this section we are concerned with the relations between fertility rates, during a defined period, of women "subsequently fertile" and the intervals between births that occur within this defined period or straddle its limits. By the term "subsequently fertile," we mean that these women give birth some time after the end of the defined period [see Chapter One, pp. 12–14].

Consider a woman with *at least* two births during such a period of length ω.[5] This period can be divided into at least three parts: the part between the start of the period ω and the first conception or birth following it; the interval between this conception and the next, then the subsequent intervals within this period; and finally, the part between the last conception within the period ω and the end of the period ω. We shall call these parts respectively the right fraction (of the straddling interval), the interior intervals, and the left fraction (of the straddling interval).[6]

---

[5] [It is assumed here that the period of time considered is sufficiently long after marriage for at least one birth to occur before the beginning of the period ω.]

[6] [When an interval between two events, say two births, straddles a certain point, say the beginning of the period (ω), let us call, on the author's suggestion, the "left" fraction of the interval the part from its beginning to the point (beginning of ω), and the "right" fraction, the part from the point (beginning of ω) to the end of the interval. As an illustration, take a woman with three births within the period ω, as follows:

	Straddling Interval			Interior Interval	Interior Interval		Straddling Interval		
	Left fraction	Right fraction					Left fraction	Right fraction	
		v		j_1	j_2		r		
1st birth			2nd birth	3rd birth		4th birth		5th birth	

beginning of ω end of ω

In the original, the "right" fraction was called "fraction avant" and the left one, "fraction arrière"; these resemble the definitions, in renewal theory, of forward and backward recurrence times respectively.]

Let us designate these several intervals by v, j_1, j_2, ..., r and let n be the number of births in the period ω. We then have

$$\omega = v + j_1 + j_2 + \ldots + j_{n-1} + r.$$

If there is only one birth, there is no interior interval and we therefore have $\omega = v + r$.

If f is the fertility rate, in this age period, of a group of k women who subsequently have at least one birth, and if the number who never conceive in the period is negligible, we then have, where n_i is the number of children borne in the period by woman i:

$$f = \frac{\sum_i n_i}{k\omega}. \tag{48}$$

The denominator $k\omega$ may also be written as:

$$k\omega = k\bar{v} + \bar{j}\Sigma(n_i - 1) + k\bar{r}, \tag{49}$$

where $\bar{v}$, $\bar{j}$, and $\bar{r}$ represent the means of v, j, and r.

We will examine these means for the case where the fundamental functions are independent of the woman's age. In that case, the distribution of an interval between two conceptions is invariant. Let $h(x)$ be its density and $H(x)$ the probability that the interval will exceed the value x. Define $\bar{i}_\omega$ as in Eq. (28) and put

$$\mu'_2 = \int_0^\infty x^2 \, h(x) \, dx \tag{50}$$

and

$$\mu'_{2\omega} = \frac{\displaystyle\int_\omega^\infty (x - \omega)^2 \, h(x) \, dx}{\displaystyle\int_\omega^\infty h(x) \, dx} = \frac{\displaystyle\int_\omega^\infty (x - \omega)^2 \, h(x) \, dx}{H(\omega)}. \tag{51}$$

We then have the following relations (which will be used subsequently);

$$dH = -h\,dx \tag{52}$$

$$\int_0^\omega h\,dx = 1 - h(\omega) \tag{53}$$

$$\int_0^\omega xhdx = \int_0^\infty xhdx - \int_\omega^\infty xhdx = \bar{\imath} - (\omega + \bar{\imath}_\omega)\, H(\omega)$$

$$(54)$$

$$\int_0^\omega x^2 hdx = \mu'_2 - H(\omega)\left[\omega^2 + \mu'_{2\omega} + 2\omega\bar{\imath}_\omega\right].$$ $$(55)$$

Also, integrating by parts:

$$\int_0^\omega Hdx = \omega\, H(\omega) + \int_0^\omega xhdx = \bar{\imath} - \bar{\imath}_\omega\, H(\omega)$$

$$(56)$$

$$\int_0^\omega xHdx = \frac{\omega^2}{2} H(\omega) + \int_0^\omega \frac{x^2}{2} hdx = \frac{\mu'_2}{2} - \left[\frac{\mu'_{2\omega}}{2} + \omega\bar{\imath}_\omega\right] H(\omega).$$

$$(57)$$

Assume that we are at the beginning of the period. For any conception that occurred at a time $(x, x + dx)$ before this beginning, there are $h(x + v)\, dxdv$ conceptions which produce a right fraction (of the straddling interval) equal to $(v, v + dx)$. Suppose that the duration of marriage at that time is sufficiently long so that the early oscillations are almost fully damped; fertility is then constant. Disregarding a constant coefficient, the expected number of right fractions with a duration of $(v, v + dx)$ is then equal to:

$$dv \int_0^\infty h(x + v)\, dx = H(v)\, dv.$$ $$(58)$$

The total number of right fractions less than ω is equal to:

$$\int_0^\omega Hdv = \bar{\imath} - \bar{\imath}_\omega\, H(\omega) \qquad \text{as in (56).}$$

The total duration of all right fractions is, disregarding the same coefficient:

$$\int_0^\omega vHdv = \frac{\mu'_2}{2} - \left[\frac{\mu'_{2\omega}}{2} + \omega\bar{\imath}_\omega\right] H(\omega), \qquad \text{as in (57).}$$

Now assume that we are at the end of the period. A proportion $H(r)$ of the conceptions that occur at $\omega - r$ are the last ones in the period. The total number of left fractions therefore is:

$$\int_0^\omega Hdr \text{ and their total duration is } \int_0^\omega rHdr.$$

Hence, the mean durations of the left and right fractions are equal. [Since we have assumed that the number of women who never conceive in ω is negligible, $H(\omega)$ is also negligible, and the sum of the mean durations of right and left fractions of straddling intervals inside ω is equal to the mean value of a straddling interval. —L.H.] The period ω may therefore be considered as consisting of n_i intervals, $n_i - 1$ interior intervals and 1 straddling interval. The quantity $\frac{k\omega}{\Sigma n_i}$ which is the inverse of the fertility rate [see Eq. (48)], is then equal to the mean value of these n_i intervals. $v + r$ is also, on the average, the half-sum of the intervals straddling the lower and the upper limit. Letting $\bar{y}$ be the mean of the straddling intervals. We have:

$$\frac{1}{f} = \frac{\bar{y}k/2 + \bar{j}\Sigma \, (n_i - 1) + \bar{y}k/2}{\Sigma n_i} \tag{59}$$

In this form, the relation in Eq. (59) shows that the inverse of the fertility rate is equal to the weighted mean of the intervals beginning or ending in the period, where the interior intervals are given twice the weight of the straddling interval.

This result can also be expressed as follows: *The fertility rate of women subsequently fertile is equal to the inverse of the mean of all intervals beginning or ending within this period; in that mean, the interior intervals intervene twice, once at their beginning and once at their end.*

To this point, we assumed simply that the fundamental functions for any woman were invariant but we have not been compelled, even implicitly, to assume that the sample was homogeneous. The result therefore applies directly to the populations investigated, provided we can assume the constancy of the fundamental functions, at least during a time interval sufficiently long on either side of the period ω (in practice, a five-year or ten-year age group).

The fertility considered is that of women *subsequently fertile:* we should also eliminate those who have had no births in the five-year period under consideration: actually, their number will probably be negligible in the case of perfect data.[7]

It will appear below, in an example, that this rule extends, as

---

[7] The omissions must in fact be responsible for a large proportion of the cases where a woman, subsequently fertile, has apparently remained infertile during one whole age group.

a perfectly adequate approximation, to cases where the fundamental functions vary with the woman's age.

Let us return now to the calculation of $\bar{v}$ and $\bar{r}$. Letting γ and γ_ω respectively be the coefficients of variation of the distribution of the intervals, starting at the beginning or after ω, we write:

$$\mu'_2 = \bar{\imath}^2(1 + \gamma^2) \tag{60}$$

$$\mu'_{2\omega} = \bar{\imath}^2{}_\omega(1 + \gamma^2{}_\omega) \tag{61}$$

and therefore, from Eq. (56) and (57):

$$\bar{v} = \bar{r} = \frac{\dfrac{\bar{\imath}^2(1 + \gamma^2)}{2} - \left[\dfrac{\bar{\imath}_\omega}{2}(1 + \gamma^2{}_\omega) + \omega\right]\bar{\imath}_\omega H(\omega)}{\bar{\imath} - \bar{\imath}_\omega H(\omega)}. \tag{62}$$

In the absence of birth control, we observe almost no intervals longer than five years; the terms in $H(\omega)$ are, therefore, negligible and we can write:

$$\bar{y} = \bar{v} + \bar{r} \approx \bar{\imath}(1 + \gamma^2). \tag{63}$$

The difference $\bar{y} - \bar{\imath}$ increases with increasing variance of the interval between two births or two conceptions. In a real, heterogeneous group, this variance results both from the variation of intervals for one woman and from the variation of the characteristics between women.

The average value $\bar{\jmath}$ of the interior intervals is given by:

$$\bar{\jmath} = \frac{\omega - \bar{y}}{f_\omega - 1} = \frac{\omega - \bar{\imath}(1 + \gamma^2)}{f_\omega - 1}. \tag{64}$$

For a homogeneous group, we furthermore have $f = 1/\bar{\imath}$ and therefore:

$$\bar{\jmath} \approx \bar{\imath}\left(1 - \frac{\bar{\imath}\gamma^2}{\omega - \bar{\imath}}\right). \tag{65}$$

The difference $\bar{y} - \bar{\jmath}$ is then equal to:

$$\bar{y} - \bar{\jmath} = \bar{\imath}\frac{\omega}{\omega - \bar{\imath}}\gamma^2. \tag{66}$$

EXAMPLES

The only available examples are furnished by historical data on families of Geneva (Henry [3]) and by the population of Crulai

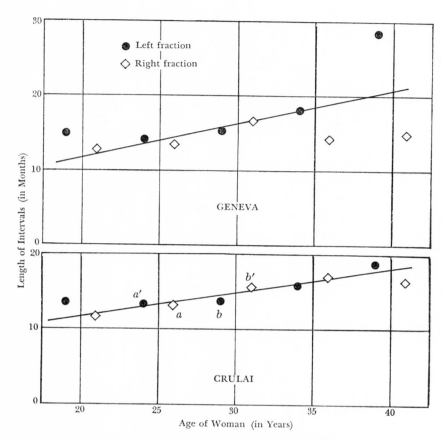

Figure 2. Left and right fractions of the straddling interval. Note: the representative points have been shifted ahead or beyond by one year which is the approximate value of the mean of the fractions of interval. The notations *a* and *a'* serve to identify certain fractions that will be discussed later.

(Gautier and Henry [1]). However, the number of observations is small, particularly for Geneva, where we prefer to restrict ourselves to the earliest period (husband born before 1600), because some features of the subsequent period (husband born in 1600 to 1649) might, if strictly interpreted, indicate the first signs of birth control. Table 1 and Figure 2 show the fractions of intervals in months at various ages of the woman.

Up to age 30, the two series resemble each other: at age 20, the left fraction is longer than the right; at 25 the difference between the two fractions is negligible; at 30, the left fraction is

TABLE 1

LENGTH (IN MONTHS) OF THE LEFT AND RIGHT FRACTION OF
INTERVALS STRADDLING SOME SPECIFIC AGES OF THE WOMEN,
FOR GENEVA AND CRULAI

	Age of Woman									
	20 years		25 years		30 years		35 years		40 years	
	fraction		fraction		fraction		fraction		fraction	
	left	right	left	right	left	right	left	right	left	right
Geneva (husband born before 1600)	14.3	12.7	14.2	13.3	15.2	16.6	18.2	14.2	28.4	14.8
No. of observations		8		22		27		23		13
Crulai (marriages of 1674-1742)	13.5	11.5	13.3	13.1	13.7	15.6	15.8	17.0	18.7	16.3
No. of observations		12		61		90		75		47

shorter than the right. At Crulai, this is still true at age 35, whereas, at Geneva, the right fraction is less at this age than the left one. At age 40, the same is true in both populations, but the difference between the two interval fractions is small at Crulai where the observations are relatively numerous, and very large in Geneva where the number is small.

The interpretation of these results is straightforward. At age 20, the observations involve very small numbers. The difference may be due to chance; otherwise, it means that fertility is lower before age 20 than later, even for fertile women. In other words, "adolescent sterility" would not be due, or not solely due, to a temporary sterility extending over a longer or shorter period after puberty. Either fecundability or the duration of the non-susceptible period would vary progressively with age, even after the first birth.

The equality of the two fractions at age 25 implies that, at about this age, the fundamental functions (fecundability, duration of the nonsusceptible period, frequency of abortion and still-birth) vary little with age. This is already known, because the fertility of women subsequently fertile is nearly the same at ages 20–24 and 25–29.

Beyond this latter age, i.e. at 30–34 and later, the fertility of

TABLE 2

LENGTH (IN MONTHS) OF THE INTERIOR AND STRADDLING
INTERVALS BETWEEN BIRTHS OCCURRING IN THE COURSE OF AGE
GROUPS 25–29 AND 30–34, FOR GENEVA AND CRULAI

	25–29 Years				30–34 Years			
	Intervals				Intervals			
	Strad-dling 25 yrs	Interior	Strad-dling 30 yrs	Weighted mean	Strad-dling 30 yrs	Interior	Strad-dling 35 yrs	Weighted mean
Geneva								
Mean of the intervals (months)	26.9	24.8	31.8	26.8	31.8	27.3	31.8	29.7
No. of intervals	21	27	21	48	23	21	23	44
Crulai								
Mean of the intervals (months)	27.2	23.0	30.6	25.4	29.6	25.9	33.0	28.5
No. of intervals	51	73	51	124	65	70	65	135

women subsequently fertile begins to decrease. As a result, the left fraction of the interval is usually shorter than the right one, since the latter corresponds to higher ages than the former.

However, when we approach the ages at which, as a rule, definitive sterility commonly begins, it becomes impossible for the right fraction to be very large. This tends to reduce its mean, until it becomes lower than the mean of the left fraction.

Let us turn now, for women having children in at least three successive age groups, to the values of the staddling and interior intervals for the age groups 25–29 and 30–34 years, as shown in Table 2.

Let us define a mean straddling interval for an age group as the arithmetic mean of the intervals that straddle its lower and upper limits. As an example, for the age group 25–29 in the Geneva data, the mean straddling interval is: $\frac{26.9 + 31.8}{2} = 29.35$. The mean difference between the straddling interval and the interior interval is 4.5 months for Geneva, and 5.4 to 5.9 months for Crulai. The relative value of these differences is appreciable, and we would make a considerable error by substituting either a

TABLE 3

FERTILITY RATE CALCULATED DIRECTLY COMPARED WITH THE
INVERSE OF THE WEIGHTED MEAN INTERVAL, FOR AGE GROUPS
25–29 AND 30–34 IN GENEVA AND CRULAI

		25–29 Years	30–34 Years
Geneva	Fertility rate	0.457	0.383
	Inverse of mean interval	0.448	0.404
Crulai	Fertility rate	0.486	0.416
	Inverse of mean interval	0.472	0.421

straddling or an interior interval for the weighted mean of the two.[8]

The data in Table 2 make it possible to calculate directly the fertility rate of women subsequently fertile, by dividing the number of births by five times the number of women. In this way, for the women in Crulai at ages 25–29, the annual fertility rate is equal to $\frac{51 + 73}{5 \times 51} = 0.486$.

Now consider the inverse of the weighted mean calculated as described above; for example, the weighted mean for Crulai at ages 25–29 is:

$$\frac{(51 \times 27.2) + (2 \times 73 \times 23.0) + (51 \times 30.6)}{51 + (2 \times 73) + 51} = 25.4$$

The inverse of this weighted mean interval expressed in years is equal to: $\frac{12}{25.4} = 0.472$.

Following the same procedure in the three other cases, we obtain the results in Table 3.

On the whole, the fertility rate and the inverse of the weighted mean interval agree well, even though the conditions for applying the theory are not strictly fulfilled: first, because the time since marriage is not sufficient for the early oscillations to become fully attenuated, and also because the fundamental functions vary with age, starting at least at age 30.

---

[8] The method of observation of intervals between births does not lend itself to a substitution of this type. This is not the case when we carry out retrospective observations. The interval elapsed between an event and an inquiry is always a left fraction of a straddling interval; this is the case, for example, for the interval elapsed since the last menstruation. Twice its mean value is greater than the mean length of the menstrual cycle. Age is also a left fraction, i.e. of the length of life, which is an interval between birth and death; twice the mean age of a stationary population is consequently always greater than the life expectancy.

This agreement cannot be considered as a result of chance. On the contrary, chance here has a rather disturbing effect. According to Figure 2, the points representing the successive fractions, whether left or right, very nearly follow a straight line from a little below age 25 to a little over age 35. If this alignment were perfect, the sum of the right and left fractions (*a* and *b* in Figure 2), belonging to the same age group would equal the sum of the complementary fractions (*a′* and *b′* in Figure 2), enclosing the same age group. Consequently, the fertility rate and the inverse of the mean interval would be equal. This is not the case because the alignment is only approximate, but we may assume that it would be better with more data.

Numerical Applications

The formulas established for the discrete process permit all desired numerical applications to be made. In principle, these formulas would make it possible to study a number of problems, unapproachable by other means, in those cases where the applicable equations cannot be solved in a manageable analytical form. In practice, this would require electronic computers. Lacking such facilities, only a few trials can be attempted and even then the lengthly calculations involved often make considerable simplification necessary.

The first simplification is to substitute the quarter for the month as the time unit used. It has been necessary also, in most cases, to forego considering variations in nonsusceptible periods, and, in most numerical applications, to assume a constant value for *g*. Finally, it has not been possible to vary the numerical data much. For example, we have considered only one maximum value of fecundability, between ages β and γ: that corresponding to the monthly value of 20 percent used in Chapter Two. On a quarterly basis it is 48.8 percent, rounded to 50 percent.[9]

---

[9] If fecundability (per month) is 20 percent, there is a 48.8 percent chance of conceiving during the first three months. This quarterly value, associated with values of K pertaining to the last month of each quarter, gives a close approximation to the number of conceptions per quarter derived from monthly calculations, as shown in Table 6 of Chapter Two. The central fertility rate calculated on this quarterly basis is, however, lower than it should be. To obtain the same value, it would have been necessary to use 50 percent as the fecundability per quarter. We have, however, retained 48.8 percent in an example, since the calculations were already well advanced before we realized that a value of 50 percent would have been preferable.

TABLE 4

PROBABILITY OF STILL BEING NONSUSCEPTIBLE FOR SPECIFIED
VALUES OF $x - \xi$ (IN QUARTERS)[1]

$x - \xi$	K	K_v	K_a	$x - \xi$	K	K_v	K_a	$x - \xi$	K	K_v	K_a
1	0.99	1	0.90	5	[0.74]	0.822	——	9	0.19	0.211	——
2	0.90	1	0.00	6	0.71	0.789	——	10	0.04	0.044	——
3	0.90	1	——	7	0.65	0.722	——	11	0.00	0.00	——
4	0.77	0.856	——	8	0.45	0.500	——	12	0.00	0.00	——

[1] This table is derived from Table 4, Chapter Two.

FIRST APPLICATION

CONCEPTIONS AND LIVE BIRTHS
ACCORDING TO ORDER

The assumptions are: fecundability is constant at a level of 0.488 for quarters 1–60 inclusive; then it decreases almost linearly to reach zero at quarter 80. This corresponds roughly to a woman marrying at, say, age 25 with fecundability at a plateau until age 40, who would become sterile at age 45 after a decrease in fecundability taking five years between age 40 and age 45.

The average duration of nonsusceptibility is 6.3 quarters or approximately nineteen months. The values of K corresponding to specified values of $x - \xi$ in quarters are shown in Table 4. Pregnancy wastage is constant and equal to 10 percent.

Table 5 shows the distribution of 10,000 women after five, ten, fifteen, and twenty years of marriage, according to the number of conceptions (A and V) and the number of V conceptions. In addition, the distribution of the number of V conceptions at the end of four years and three months is given, as equivalent to the distribution of live births at the end of five years of marriage.

As long as fecundability is constant, say up to fifteen years of marriage, the mean number of conceptions is approximately proportional to marital duration plus nine months. The ratio equals the average annual fertility rate, either total (conceptions), or effective (live-births).

Variation here is due to chance alone. We are dealing, by assumption, with a homogeneous group, and differences between members of this group arise from the random nature of conception, of the outcome of pregnancy and of variations in the duration of nonsusceptibility.

TABLE 5

DISTRIBUTION OF 10,000 WOMEN ACCORDING TO THE CUMULATIVE
NUMBER OF CONCEPTIONS (C) AND OF CONCEPTIONS OF
LIVE-BORN CHILDREN (V) AT THE CONCLUSION OF DIFFERENT
DURATIONS OF MARRIAGE

Number of Conceptions	Duration of Marriage									
	4 years 3 months	5 years		10 years		15 years		20 years		
	V	C	V	C	V	C	V	C	V
0	1	——	——	——	——	——	——	——	——
1	553	32	135	——	——	——	——	——	——
2	7,474	3,703	5,253	——	3	——	——	——	——
3	1,983	5,139	4,378	63	300	——	——	——	——
4	39	1,029	232	2,123	4,009	1	10	——	——
5	——	92	2	4,801	4,793	68	402	1	12
6	——	5	——	2,394	852	1,331	3,261	46	298
7	——	——	——	539	43	3,818	4,596	671	2,083
8	——	——	——	73	——	3,181	1,551	2,575	4,193
9	——	——	——	7	——	1,251	172	3,459	2,681
10	——	——	——	——	——	296	8	2,195	658
11	——	——	——	——	——	48	——	812	71
12	——	——	——	——	——	6	——	200	4
13	——	——	——	——	——	——	——	36	——
14	——	——	——	——	——	——	——	5	——
Total	10,000	10,000	10,000	10,000	10,000	10,000	10,000	10,000	10,000
Mean no. conceptions	2.1556	2.7461	2.4713	5.1470	4.632	7.5323	6.7824	9.0530	8.1511
Variance	0.240	0.463	0.324	0.748	0.492	1.055	0.680	1.280	0.917
Standard deviation	0.490	0.680	0.569	0.865	0.701	1.027	0.824	1.131	0.958
Coefficient of variation	0.227	0.247	0.230	0.168	0.151	0.136	0.122	0.125	0.117

The absolute variation increases with the number of conceptions, but less rapidly; so that the relative variation, measured by the coefficient of variation (the ratio of the standard deviation to the mean) decreases as the mean increases. The variance is roughly proportional to the mean.

For equivalent mean values, the relative variation of live births is less than that of conceptions.

Although the coefficient of variation is low for long durations of marriage, the variation is far from negligible; 2 or 3 values of

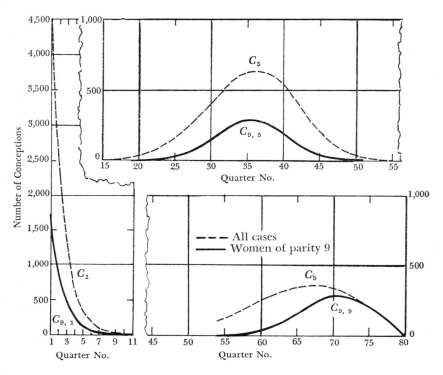

Figure 3. Distribution of conceptions of order 1, 5, and 9, for all cases (C_1, C_5, and C_9) and for women with completed parity equal to 9 ($C_{9,1}$, $C_{9,5}$ and $C_{9,9}$).

family size are relatively important; and 3 or 4 are non-negligible. But the variation is clearly less marked than that observed in real and necessarily heterogeneous populations. At Crulai, for example, the coefficient of variation of the number of live births of complete families with at least one child is 0.34 for women married at 25 (6.17 births per mother on the average) and 0.32 for women married at age 20 (8.15 births per mother on the average).

Table 6 shows the distribution, for the 3,459 hypothetical women who had nine conceptions, of the time at which they experienced conceptions Nos. 1, 5, and 9. Figure 3, which illustrates this table, clearly shows the differences in the variation of the time for all conceptions of a certain order and of the time for conceptions of the same order in families with exactly nine conceptions.

TABLE 6

DISTRIBUTION OF TIME OF CONCEPTIONS OF ORDER 1, 5, AND 9 IN FAMILIES WITH 9 CONCEPTIONS

Order 1

Quarters No.	C_1	$P_{8,c}$ per 1000	$C_{9,1}$
1	4,880	351	1,713
2	2,500	350	874
3	1,279	345	441
4	655	336	220
5	335	325	109
6	172	310	53
7	88	293	26
8	45	273	12
9	25	253	6
10	12	231	3
11	6	209	1
12	3	187	—
13	2	166	—
14	1	146	—
Total	3,459		

Order 5

Quarters No.	C_5	$P_{4,c}$ per 1000	$C_{9,5}$
10	—	—	—
11	—	—	—
12	1	4	—
13	1	6	—
14	2	8	—
15	4	12	—
16	9	17	—
17	10	24	—
18	16	32	—
19	23	43	1
20	34	57	2
21	48	75	4
22	66	96	6
23	89	120	11
24	118	149	18
25	154	180	28
26	196	215	42
27	243	252	61
28	293	289	85
29	345	326	113
30	401	361	145
31	460	393	181
32	517	419	217
33	567	439	248
34	604	451	272
35	625	455	284
36	633	450	285
37	629	438	275
38	612	418	256
39	582	392	228
40	536	361	194
41	477	326	156
42	407	290	118
43	335	253	85
44	266	216	57
45	204	181	37
46	152	149	23
47	110	121	13
48	78	96	7
49	59	74	4
50	37	57	2
51	24	42	1
52	16	31	—
53	10	22	—
54	7	15	—
55	4	10	—
56	3	7	—
57	2	4	—
58	1	3	—
59	1	2	—
Total	3,459		

Order 9

Quarters No.	C_9	$P_{0,c}$ per 1000	$C_{9,9}$
54	102	8	1
55	122	14	2
56	144	23	3
57	169	37	6
58	196	56	11
59	224	83	19
60	254	118	30
61	277	164	45
62	294	219	64
63	311	285	89
64	328	360	118
65	341	442	151
66	350	528	185
67	356	615	219
68	356	697	248
69	351	772	271
70	339	835	283
71	322	884	284
72	299	919	275
73	273	945	258
74	243	966	235
75	211	982	207
76	175	992	174
77	136	997	136
78	95	1,000	95
79	50	1,000	50
Total	3,459		

Note: C_k is the distribution of kth conceptions regardless of completed fertility (not all of the conceptions of the respective order are shown). $P_{k,c}$ is as defined in Eq. (45) and $C_{9,k} = C_k \, P_{9-k,c}$.

93

TABLE 7

DISTRIBUTION OF 10,000 COMPLETE FAMILIES BY THE NUMBER
OF BIRTHS WITH DECLINING AND WITH CONSTANT FECUNDABILITY

Number of Births	Declining Fecundability from 61st to 80th Quarter	Duration in Quarters Fecundability Constant				
		71	72	73	74	75
7	53	40	25	15	9	5
8	892	1,010	733	523	368	256
9	4,323	5,806	5,170	4,463	3,743	3,058
10	4,273	3,139	4,041	4,887	5,594	6,090
11	459	5	31	112	286	591
Total	10,000	10,000	10,000	10,000	10,000	10,000
Mean no. of children	9.42	9.21	9.33	9.46	9.58	9.70

OTHER APPLICATIONS

Because of the lengthy calculations involved, the following results were obtained from simplified models with a constant nonsusceptible period and without pregnancy wastage.

EFFECTS OF DECLINE IN FECUNDABILITY

Consider first a group in which fecundability, constant and
equal to 0.5 per quarter until the 60th quarter, thereafter falls
linearly, to reach zero in the 80th quarter. For a constant nonsusceptible period of 6 quarters the distribution of 10,000 complete families, according to the number of births, is shown in
Table 7. Let us see to what extent the same result could be obtained
with the same nonsusceptible period and a fecundability of 0.5
per quarter maintained from the beginning to the end of a period
appreciably shorter than 80 quarters.[10] If we consider only the
mean number of births, 73 quarters is the "equivalent" to the real
duration of fecundity, i.e. 79 quarters. But the distribution is not
the same; there is less variation with constant fecundability. For better approximations, it would be necessary simultaneously to modify both fecundability and the nonsusceptible period. By decreasing both together while keeping central fertility constant, one
would increase the variation. To put it another way, efforts to fit
models where fecundability does not decrease towards the end of

---

[10] This problem arises in relation to the research of W. Brass [1].

TABLE 8

MEAN DURATION OF MARRIAGE (IN QUARTERS) AT DELIVERY, BY
BIRTH ORDER FOR THE TOTAL, FOR LAST BIRTHS, AND
OTHER BIRTHS OF ORDER 7 THROUGH 11

	Birth Order				
	7	8	9	10	11
	Mean Duration of Marriage				
Total	50.00	57.97	65.42	70.48	72.68
Last births	65.57	66.79	68.33	70.59	72.68
Others	49.98	57.49	62.83	65.52	———

the fecund period run the risk of underestimating both fecundability and the duration of nonsusceptibility.

INTERVALS BETWEEN BIRTHS

Let us first consider the model without a decrease in fecundability. To calculate the mean interval between, say, the eighth and ninth births, it is necessary to calculate the mean duration of marriage at the time of the ninth birth and subtract from it the mean duration of marriage at the time of the eighth births *which are not the last*. These durations appear in Table 8, which also shows the mean duration of marriage at the birth of the last child of each birth order. The interval between the eighth and ninth births is obtained by subtracting 57.49 from 65.42 which gives 7.93 quarters.

Similar calculations for other birth-orders and conversion to months, yield the following results:

1–2 to 6–7	7–8	8–9	9–10	10–11
24	23.97	23.79	22.95	21.48 .

Thus, intervals between births decrease although the "aptitude," is, by assumption, invariant throughout the period under consideration. The group is, moreover, assumed to be homogeneous. *One would, therefore, commit a serious error of interpretation in attributing this decline in interval lengths either to a modification of the aptitudes or to selection of the most fecund women as birth order increases.*

In the homogeneous group on which the calculations were made, all families have at least seven births; but a few stop at seven, while others go further, a few achieving eleven births. This differentiation, *due to chance and to chance alone,* is associated

TABLE 9

MEAN INTERVALS BETWEEN BIRTHS BY SIZE
OF THE COMPLETE FAMILY

Size of the Complete Family	Mean Interval (Months)
7	29.25
8	27.00
9	24.80
10	23.00
11	21.50

with differences in the intervals between births. In each category of complete family size, the mean interval between births is the same, regardless of order. But this mean interval varies with the size of the complete family as shown in Table 9.

Let us return to the interval between the eighth and ninth births. Relevant data are available in 9,462 hypothetical families. Of these, 4,463 families stop at nine births and have a mean interval of 24.8 months; 4,887 stop at ten and have a mean interval of 23.0; 112 stop at eleven and have a mean interval of 21.5.

We have, then:

$$23.8 = \frac{24.8 \times 4,463 + 23.0 \times 4,887 + 21.5 \times 112}{9,462}.$$

In other words, the mean interval between births n and $n + 1$ is a weighted mean of the mean intervals in families of size $n + 1$, $n + 2$, $n + 3$ and so on. As long as the proportion of families with fewer than $n + 1$ births is negligible, this weighted mean is constant; when this is no longer the case, *the mean diminishes as* n *increases, since families with longer mean intervals are progressively eliminated.*

From the same model, the mean marital duration for births of each order, in months, is as in Table 10.

In a group of complete families *of the same size,* the difference between two successive mean marital durations is equal to the mean interval between births of the corresponding order. This is true in Table 10 for births or order 7 and below, *achieved by practically all the families.* Beyond seven births, the difference decreases, even more rapidly than does the mean interval. This is so because women who have, say, their eighth child late in life are those that also have the least chance of having a ninth birth.

Thus, chance alone produces, in a homogeneous group, phenomena analogous to those observed in real, heterogeneous

TABLE 10

MEAN DURATION OF MARRIAGE (IN MONTHS) AT DELIVERY BY
BIRTH ORDER AND DIFFERENCE IN THE DURATION BETWEEN
TWO SUCCESSIVE ORDERS

Order	Mean Duration of Marriage	Difference from the Preceding
1	13.5	——
2	37.5	24.0
3	61.5	24.0
4	85.5	24.0
5	109.5	24.0
6	133.5	24.0
7	157.5	24.0
8	181.4	23.9
9	203.8	22.4
10	218.9	15.1
11	225.5	6.6

groups. From this result we may draw a practical and prudent conclusion: *differentiation between real families is due both to differences in aptitude and to chance; it would be dangerous to interpret it as a consequence of differences in aptitude only.*

INFLUENCE ON INTERVALS BETWEEN BIRTHS
OF A PROGRESSIVE DECREASE IN FECUNDABILITY
WITH THE WOMAN'S AGE

Study of populations generally considered not to practice birth control shows that on the average the interval to the last birth is longer than the earlier intervals. Some demographers have seen in this a sign of birth control. In fact it does often happen that an unwanted last conception occurs after a long period of continence or successful contraception.

But it also is reasonable to think that fecundability diminishes towards the end of the reproductive period, because sexual intercourse is less frequent, or because anovular cycles or very early abortions are more frequent. We should therefore inquire to what extent a decline in fecundability can bring about an increase in the mean interval between births.

Here also, we content ourselves with a greatly simplified model with an invariant period of nonsusceptibility; but we have used three different values for the duration of the nonsusceptible period. Initial fecundability was put at 0.500 in all cases; but the linear decline to zero was spread over either five years, ten years,

TABLE 11

CHARACTERISTIC INTERVAL BETWEEN BIRTHS AND MEANS OF
SPECIFIED INTERVALS COUNTING FROM THE END FOR
THREE DURATIONS OF FECUNDABILITY DECLINE

Duration of Fecundability Decline	Length of Nonsusceptible Period (Quarters)	Interval (in Months)				
		Characteristic Interval	Preceding Antepenultimate (L − 3)	Antepenultimate (L − 2)	Penultimate (L − 1)	Last (L)
5 years	6	24.00	24.00	24.00	24.36	27.33
	8	30.00	30.00	30.00	30.00	32.88
	10	36.00	36.00	36.00	36.03	38.46
10 years	6	24.00	24.15	25.02	27.15	31.77
	8	30.00	30.03	30.45	32.34	37.23
	10	36.00	——	36.15	37.71	42.66
15 years	6	24.00	25.50	27.03	29.70	35.25
	8	30.00	——	32.25	34.86	40.62
	10	36.00	——	37.53	40.11	46.05

Note: The characteristic interval is equal to the sum of the nonsusceptible period and of the inverse of fecundability. Thus, $6 + \frac{1}{0.5} = 8$ quarters $= 24$ months.

or fifteen years in the three cases. Three values of the nonsusceptible period and three rates of decline in fecundability yield nine combinations, requiring lengthy calculations.

Table 11 gives mean intervals (in months) between births, obtained for births counted from the end regardless of completed fertility.

If the differences between the mean interval and the characteristic interval are illustrated graphically (Figure 4), we find that there is relatively little difference, within each category of fecundability decline, between results corresponding to diverse values of the nonsusceptible period. In what follows, we will therefore use a single mean value of 8 quarters.

We observe the following: if the decline in fecundability is rapid, lengthening occurs only in the last interval and amounts to only about three months. If the decline is spread over twice as much time (ten years), an appreciable increase is noted even in the second last interval. The total increase, i.e. the difference between the length of the last interval and that of the characteristic interval, exceeds six months. Finally, if we postulate a linear

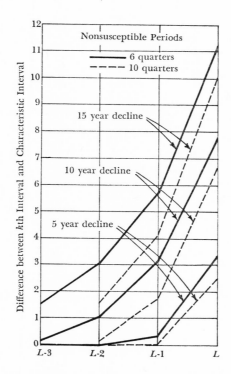

Figure 4. Lengthening of intervals where L is last interval, L-1 second last, etc., according to duration of decline in fecundability toward end of reproductive period.

decrease taking fifteen years, the last three intervals are increased in length and the total increase exceeds ten months.

The calculations were made with only one value of fecundability. This value corresponds, by and large, to the average value at the beginning of marriage as observed at Geneva and Crulai in women married between ages 20 and 29.

What would happen if fecundability were one half as great? In the continuous case, to say that fecundability is half as great is the same as saying that the mean number of conceptions is equal to pdt, during an interval of time equal to $2dt$ instead of to dt. It follows that by taking a time unit twice as long, we have the same equations and, therefore, the same numerical results with $(p/2, 2g)$ as with (p, g).[11] Expressed in the same time units,

---

[11] [See Eqs. (7) and (8) in Chapter One.]

TABLE 12

DIFFERENCE (IN QUARTERS) BETWEEN THE LAST INTERVAL AND THE
CHARACTERISTIC INTERVAL FOR SPECIFIED COMBINATIONS OF
FECUNDABILITY, DURATION OF FECUNDABILITY DECLINE, AND
DURATION OF NONSUSCEPTIBILITY

[Fecundability] per Quarter before Decline	Duration of Decline (yrs)	Nonsusceptible Period (Quarters)	Characteristic Interval (Quarters)	Last Interval (Quarters)	Lengthening (Quarters)
0.25	10	8	12	14.54	2.54
0.50	5	4	6	(7.26)	1.26

Note: The value (7.26) quarters is the result of a linear extrapolation in Table 11, calculated as follows: $\dfrac{27.33 - (32.88 - 27.33)}{3} = 7.26$.

the results given by $(p/2, 2g)$, are double those of (p, g). Thus, the lengthening in the last interval observed in forty years of marriage with a stated fecundability, a fecundability decline taking twenty years, and a nonsusceptible period of twenty-four months, will be double that observed in twenty years of marriage with a doubled fecundability, a decline taking ten years, and a nonsusceptible period of twelve months.

If the reduction in fecundability begins only after a fairly long duration of marriage, fertility is almost stabilized at the beginning of this reduction. The time elapsed since marriage is of practically no importance. The same holds true for total marital duration. Hence, we obtain the following version of the above result: the increase in the last interval corresponding to a specific fecundability, with a reduction over twenty years and a nonsusceptible period of twenty-four months, is twice as great as that corresponding to a fecundability twice as high, a reduction over ten years, and a nonsusceptible period of twelve months.

In the discrete case, the relationship between $(p/2, 2g)$ and (p, g) remains, but it does not have exactly the same meaning as in the continuous case. Though expressed in different units, we get the same numerical results with:

$p = 0.5$ per quarter $g = 4$ quarters
$p = 0.5$ half-yearly $g = 4$ half-years or 8 quarters,

but a fecundability of 0.5 per half-year is not equivalent, in all respects, to one of 0.25 per quarter. We must, therefore, revert to numerical calculation to see how the increase in the last interval takes place. The results, in quarters, are shown in Table 12.

TABLE 13

LENGTHENING (IN QUARTERS) IN THE LAST INTERVAL BY DURATION
OF THE FECUNDABILITY DECLINE FOR TWO LEVELS OF
FECUNDABILITY

[Fecundability] per Quarter before Decline	Duration of Decline			
	5 years	10 years	15 years	20 years
	Lengthening in Quarters			
0.25	——	2.54	[4.04]	5.54
0.50	[0.96]	2.41	3.54	——

Note: $0.96 = \dfrac{32.88 - 30.00}{3}$, $2.41 = \dfrac{37.23 - 30.00}{3}$, $3.54 = \dfrac{40.62 - 30.00}{3}$. The values 4.04 and 5.54 were obtained by extrapolation as explained in Table 12 and the results were multiplied by 2 to adjust for the value of fecundability equal to 0.25 instead of 0.50.

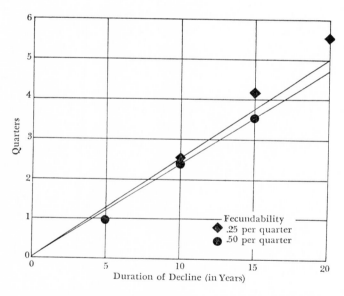

Figure 5. Lengthening of last interval, by quarter and value of fecundability and duration of its decline.

Equivalence, *a priori* uncertain, therefore exists and we may operate as in the continuous case. For a nonsusceptible period of 8 quarters, the increase is as in Table 13, according to the duration of the decline in fecundability.

From Figure 5 we see that the lengthening is approximately

TABLE 14

MEAN OF LAST INTERVALS FOR COMPLETE FAMILIES OF SIX
CHILDREN OR MORE, FOR JAPAN, CRULAI, AND GENEVA

	Preceding Antepenultimate (L − 3)	Antepenultimate (L − 2)	Penultimate (L − 1)	Last Interval (L)
Japan	33.2	33.3	35.9	42.3
Crulai (marriages from 1674–1742)	29.1	32.0	31.9	39.7
Geneva (husband born before 1600)	29.2	28.7	33.0	39.4

proportional to the duration of the decline as long as this duration does not exceed fifteen years; and, further, that the lengthening depends little on fecundability. This last finding, moreover,
follows from the first and from the relatively unimportant effect,
already mentioned, of the length of the nonsusceptible period.

Finally, we reach the following approximate result: the positive difference between the last interval and the characteristic interval depends little on fecundability or the nonsusceptible period; it is proportional to the duration of decline (supposedly
linear) in fecundability.

For this reason, comparison of models with empirical data may
inform us about the duration of the linear decline in fecundability, which we must assume exists in order to explain actual observations by this feature. Such observations are not numerous;
the best documented relate to the agricultural population of
Japan and come from a 1940 field study of complete families
(Okasaki [1]). The disadvantage is that there is no assurance of
the total absence of birth control. Other observations, made in
Geneva and Crulai, bear on historical populations, and the number of records of complete families is unfortunately very scanty.

The mean of the last four intervals, in months, for complete
families of at least six children is given in Table 14. The incre-
ments, shown in Figure 6, are of the order of magnitude of those
obtained in the calculations made with a fecundability decline
taking from ten to fifteen years.

In the preceding, we neglected the final family size in order to
see what occurs overall toward the end of the procreative period.
Let us now reintroduce this size, limiting ourselves, as before, to
a single value for the nonsusceptible period. But we will take 6
quarters instead of 8 in order to have a more extended range

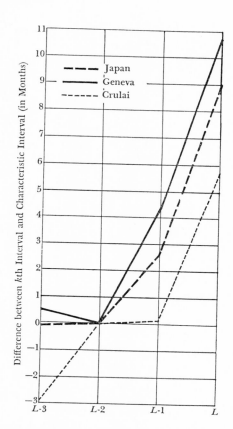

Figure 6. Lengthening of intervals where L is last, $L-1$ second last, etc., according to duration of decline in fecundability toward end of reproductive period.

of family size and birth orders in the 80 quarters to which our calculations are limited. Table 15 gives mean intervals in months and the results are illustrated in the lower part of Figure 7. A similar tabulation appears in Table 16, which shows the mean intervals between births (in months) obtained by graphic adjustment of the mean intervals observed in Japan.

The graphic translation of Table 16 (Figure 7, top) shows that the increase in intervals is actually preceded, not by a plateau, but by a slight upward slope.

This increase is almost entirely limited to the last two intervals, but it remains marked in large families. Now these two features are not seen in any one model; the first corresponds to what we

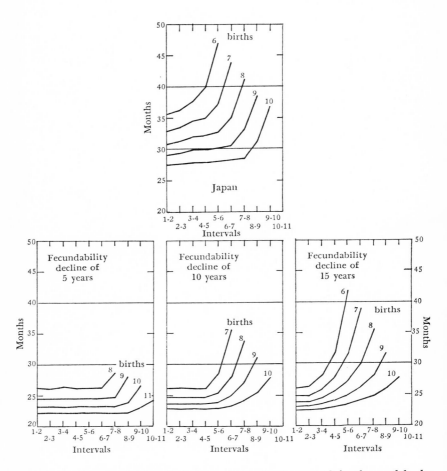

Figure 7. Length of intervals between births in Japan and in the models, by birth order, the total number of births (completed parity), and, for the models, the duration of the decline in fecundability.

might call an intermediate duration of the decline in fecundability; the second, on the contrary, to a long duration. It may be observed, moreover, that the curves of the Japanese data are much more widely separated from each other than are those of the models.

This last difference is self-explanatory. In a real population, chance is not the only reason for differences between families; they vary in the effective duration of the union (the period in which a couple can have children) and in their aptitudes (fecun-

TABLE 15

MEAN INTERVAL BETWEEN BIRTHS ACCORDING TO BIRTH
ORDER, THE NUMBER OF BIRTHS, AND THE DURATION OF THE
DECLINE IN FECUNDABILITY

Total Number of Births	Mean Interval between Births									
	1–2	2–3	3–4	4–5	5–6	6–7	7–8	8–9	9–10	10–11
Fecundability Decline of 5 years										
8	26.22	26.07	26.37	26.13	26.16	26.16	28.68	——	——	——
9	24.48	24.45	24.45	24.48	24.45	24.48	24.63	28.05	——	——
10	23.22	23.22	23.19	23.25	23.16	23.25	23.22	23.85	26.67	——
11	22.13	22.23	22.17	22.17	22.23	22.14	22.20	22.23	23.04	24.21
Fecundability Decline of 10 years										
7	26.10	26.18	26.10	26.01	28.38	35.52	——	——	——	——
8	24.66	24.69	24.66	24.66	25.32	27.93	33.87	——	——	——
9	23.64	23.64	23.61	23.64	23.79	24.96	26.97	31.14	——	——
10	22.80	22.77	22.80	22.77	22.83	23.34	24.15	25.47	27.84	——
Fecundability Decline of 15 years										
6	26.04	26.28	28.08	31.77	41.82	——	——	——	——	——
7	24.84	24.87	25.92	27.87	31.35	38.35	——	——	——	——
8	23.91	23.94	24.54	25.59	27.21	29.91	35.43	——	——	——
9	23.19	23.19	23.52	24.12	24.99	26.16	28.08	31.59	——	——
10	22.53	22.53	22.71	23.07	23.40	24.09	24.78	25.95	27.66	——

TABLE 16

ADJUSTED MEAN INTERVAL BETWEEN BIRTHS (IN MONTHS) BY
ORDER AND BY COMPLETED FERTILITY (JAPANESE DATA)

Total Number of Births	Intervals between Births								
	1–2	2–3	3–4	4–5	5–6	6–7	7–8	8–9	9–10
6	35.6	36.2	37.6	39.8	47.1	——	——	——	——
7	32.8	33.4	34.4	34.9	37.2	43.8	——	——	——
8	30.7	31.2	31.9	32.2	32.7	35.0	41.2	——	——
9	29.0	29.3	29.8	29.8	30.2	30.6	33.0	38.4	——
10	27.4	27.6	27.8	27.8	28.1	28.3	28.5	31.1	36.8

dability and nonsusceptible period). Families that have the most children are those with the longest effective durations, those whose nonsusceptible period is the shortest and, to a lesser degree, those whose fecundability is highest.

TABLE 17

DISTRIBUTION OF NUMBER OF BIRTHS PER 1,000 FAMILIES
FOR TWO DURATIONS OF FECUNDABILITY DECLINE

| | Number of Families Having the Number of Births Listed | |
| | Fecundability Decline | |
Number of Births	10 years	15 years
5 or less	—	4
6	5	48
7	66	231
8	317	422
9	455	255
10	151	39
More than 10	6	1
Total	1,000	1,000

But inequality of the effective durations cannot spread the curves.[12] The spread observed in a real population must therefore be due to inequality of aptitudes: fecundability and the nonsusceptible period. Differences in the effective duration have one other effect: families with identical aptitudes[13] and different effective durations should have fairly similar histories, on the average, during the effective duration common to them, which extends from the age at the latest marriage up to definitive sterility. Consequently, the last intervals should be the same, say, in eight-child families with a shorter effective duration as in ten-child families with a longer effective duration. Comparisons between models and reality should therefore not necessarily be limited to families of the same size.

---

[12] Let us increase the effective marital duration of half the couples by advancing marriage in such a way that there are two additional intervals. These two intervals are the same length as interval L-2 of the other half. The following values were then obtained for interval L-2 in the case where fecundability declines over fifteen years:

Family Size	Interval Size
7 children	24.84
8 children	24.12
9 children	23.94
10 children	23.80
11 children	23.19

The means corresponding to the most common family sizes vary less.

[13] Which supposes the same age at definite sterility.

TABLE 18

MEAN INTERVAL BETWEEN BIRTHS (IN MONTHS) BY COMPLETED
FERTILITY GIVEN A FECUNDABILITY DECLINE OVER TEN YEARS

Total Number of Births	Interval between Births of Order						
	3–4	4–5	5–6	6–7	7–8	8–9	9–10
8	24.9	24.9	25.4	28.0	34.2	——	——
9	——	24.1	24.1	25.1	27.4	32.3	——
10	——	——	23.4	23.7	24.7	26.6	30.4

Now, we can see that the Japanese curves for families of size 7 to 10 closely approximate (neglecting the slow rise to the second (L-2) or third (L-3) from the last), the curves of families of size 7 and 8 in the average model (decline taking ten years). For six-child families, the initial rise is steeper than for the others, but the end of the curves from the second last to the last is almost exactly the same. We do not therefore observe the kind of relationship between the number of children and the shape of the curves that is so characteristic of the models with fecundability declines taking ten and fifteen years. Everything proceeds in Japan as if the increase in the later intervals were the same for all family sizes.

In the models, differences in family size are a result of chance. The same is true, therefore, of differences between curves according to family size. Hence, the absence of such variation in Japan could mean that in reality the effects of chance are negligible and that differences in family size result only from differences in the effective durations of marriage. But in the models there is no preponderant family size; several sizes have non-negligible frequencies, as shown in Table 17, corresponding to the models of Table 15.

However, let us see if heterogeneity of effective durations might not apparently minimize the effects of chance. For that purpose, let us increase the effective durations of one-half the families in such a way that they would have one additional birth. We assume that the intervals counting from the end remain unaltered; their order is simply increased by one.

Under these conditions we have the values shown in Table 18 for the intervals in the case of a decline in fecundability taking ten years, when completed parity equals 8, 9, or 10. For these three family sizes, the most frequent, the modification in form

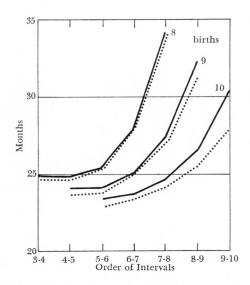

Figure 8. Last few intervals according to whether the effective durations are the same (dotted line) or not (solid line).

is in fact less pronounced than in the model, as shown in Figure 8. Nevertheless, it still exists, so that we must conclude that the models studied do not give a perfect account of the observations made in Japan.

Those observations are so far the only ones that are sufficiently numerous to permit detailed comparison with models. Let us imagine, however, that later observations of other populations with little contraceptive use produce the same findings. We would then draw the following conclusions which, in the meantime, may be considered as working hypotheses.

As long as we disregard the variations in the lengthening of the last intervals that are observed according to parity, we can explain the lengthening by a linear decline in fecundability and even estimate the order of magnitude (ten to twelve years) of the duration of this decline.

This is no longer the case if we take into account the effect of final parity on the lengthening. In the largest families the lengthening of the last intervals is more marked than in the models.

The models should therefore be modified to approach reality more closely. One might, for example, imagine that the duration of the nonsusceptible period rises progressively with the woman's age. It is to be feared, however, that this modification would lead nowhere. Indeed, it seems to us that the progression of the lengthening observed in models with a prolonged decline of fecundability would be repeated in models where the duration of the nonsusceptible period increased over an appreciable number of years. On the average, families of the largest final size will have, during those years, a larger number of births than families of a smaller final size. Hence, the number of intervals affected by the progressive change in nonsusceptible periods would be greater. It probably will be necessary to seek elsewhere.

PROBLEM PRESENTED IN MEASURING THE FERTILITY OF FECUND COUPLES

In studying the fertility of noncontracepting populations, one seeks to separate couples who are still fecund from those, increasingly more numerous with increase in the women's age, who are subsequently sterile. For families of the Geneva bourgeoisie of the historic period and for families of Crulai we adopted the approximate solution of substituting for fecund women of a given age group, 35 to 39, for example, women described as subsequently fertile, who gave birth after this age group, i.e. at age 40 and above.

We knew that this introduced a selective bias, since women bearing children after a short interval had a greater chance of being subsequently fertile than those whose confinements were more widely spaced. We considered the possible importance of this bias and concluded that it mattered little until the age of 40. But we ignored another, less obvious, bias related to the very definition of this subsequently fertile group of women. Of course, this group is defined by observations made at ages outside the age group considered (35 to 39 in the example above). But those observations would be independent of those made in the 35 to 39 age group only if no nonsusceptible period were involved, which is, of course, impossible. The reason is as follows: women who have many births between ages 35 and 39—three births for example—have the last of these births (the third) a very short time before the upper limit of the age group, their fortieth birthday. Consequently, they are often in the nonsusceptible state when they pass this age limit. Women who have only one birth between ages 35 and 39 are, on the contrary, usually not in the nonsusceptible state when they reach age 40. Hence, such women

TABLE 19

DISTRIBUTION OF NUMBER OF BIRTHS DURING FIVE YEARS

OF MARRIAGE AND SUBSEQUENT FERTILITY

(ASSUMING NO STERILITY)

Quarter	First Age Group			Second Age Group Fecundability .500			Second Age Group Fecundability .250		
	Births			Subsequent First Birth at					
	N_{11} (1)	N_{22} (2)	N_{33} (3)	N_{11} (4)	N_{22} (5)	N_{33} (6)	N_{11} (7)	N_{22} (8)	N_{33} (9)
1	1	——	——	312	688	——	156	344	——
2	1	——	——	188	812	——	133	493	——
3	2	——	——	109	891	——	107	611	——
4	4	——	——	63	938	——	85	705	——
5	8	——	——	35	965	——	65	776	——
6	16	——	——	19	980	——	50	831	——
7	31	——	——	11	989	——	38	873	——
8	62	——	——	6	869	125	29	842	62
9	125	——	——	4	684	313	22	756	172
10	125	125	——	4	342	156	16	567	129
11	125	375	——	1	170	78	12	425	97
12	125	875	——	——	86	39	9	319	73
13	62	938	——	——	43	19	7	239	55
14	31	969	——	——	21	10	5	179	41
15	16	984	——	——	11	5	4	134	31
16	8	992	——	——	6	3	3	101	23
17	4	996	——	——	2	1	2	75	17
18	2	998	——	——	1	1	2	56	13
19	1	749	250	——	——	——	1	42	10
20	1	499	500	——	——	——	1	32	8

Note: N_{11} designates births of order 1 to women having only one birth in the first age group; N_{22}, births of order 2 to women having exactly 2 births in the age group, and so on.

Cumulation of the numbers in column (4) gives the number of women in group N_{11} who, in the absence of sterility, would be subsequently fertile before the end of the first quarter of the second age group, before the end of the 2nd quarter, etc. Thus we have 672 giving birth before the end of the first year (312 + 188 + 109 + 63); 743 before the end of the second; 750 before the end of the third. [Because of rounding errors, the total is only 749 instead of 750 as in column (1). The same thing makes column (5) different from column (2). The differences between the totals of coluns (7), (8), (9) and those of columns (1), (2), (3) have a different cause: in the case of a lower fecundability, a small proportion of the women have no births in the second age group.] On the assumption that 200 women out of 1000 became sterile at the beginning of the first year of the second age group, 200 more at the beginning of the second year, and so on, the total number of women of group N_{11} who are subsequently fertile equals .8 (672) + .6 (71), etc. which is equivalent to 0.200 × 672 + 0.200 × 743 + 0.200 × 750 + 0.200 × 750 or 583; in the same way we find 5,474 for group N_{22} and 317 for have more time to bear another child before becoming sterile, and therefore a greater chance of being included in the group of subsequently fertile women. This group therefore includes too high a proportion of women who had few births between 35 and 39, and too low a proportion of women who had many. This is definitely a bias of definition that acts in the opposite direction to the selection bias, but whereas the selection bias exists only because of the heterogeneity of observable populations, the definition bias affects each component homogeneous population.

The question then arises whether this inevitable bias is serious. To ascertain this, let us consider a group in which fecundability per quarter equals 0.5 and the nonsusceptible period lasts 8 quarters. The central fertility rate is 0.1 per quarter. We assume this level has been reached before the beginning of the age group under consideration, and consequently, this level is maintained among women who remain fertile to the end of this five-year age group. We suppose further that these women become sterile during the succeeding five-year period at the following rates: 20 percent on leaving the age group, 20 percent one year later, 20 percent two years later, and so on.

The calculations (see Table 19) show that subsequently fertile women had on the average 1.96 births during the five-year period considered, whereas the average for all fecund women in the age group was two children. The selection bias is very small, although a rapid progression of sterility was assumed. The bias remains small if it is assumed that a decrease in fecundability accompanies the progression of sterility: under similar conditions in the same age group, with the same progression of sterility beyond this age, but with fecundability reduced by half, the result is 1.95 as opposed to 2.00.

Note that the definition bias is virtually eliminated if subsequently fertile women are defined as those that have at least one birth two years after the upper limit of the age group being considered, i.e. beyond age 42 for the 35–39 age group.

---

group N_{33}. The average number of children in the first age group is:

$$\frac{583 + 2 \times 5474 + 3 \times 317}{6374}, \quad \text{or } 1.96$$

To obtain the number of women fertile beyond the second year after the first age group, start with the preceding table to calculate the initial births, beginning with quarter 9, that follow those shown in columns (4) through (9) for quarters 1 through 8.

Note also that the conclusions reached through a study of five-year age groups would not be identical with those of a study by single years of age. The definition bias is no longer negligible toward the end of the reproductive period when sterility progresses very rapidly. The reason is simple: the distribution of fecund women according to the number of births in five years of conjugal life shows little dispersion. Within a one-year span, on the contrary, roughly half the women have one birth and the rest have none. This second half clearly accounts for more subsequently fertile women than the first, once the progression of sterility is rapid.

CONCLUSION

This article has not exhausted the very extensive material related to family building from marriage onward. We might, in particular, have greatly extended our study of cases in which the fundamental functions remain constant, and we might also have given other numerical applications.

But since we could not fit everything into the scope of a single article, it seemed preferable to retain general formulas rather than those applicable only to particular cases. As for numerical applications, their choice was guided by a concern to illustrate the theoretical portion of the article and by the desire to demonstrate the use of models in interpreting certain observations.

To conclude, we wish to emphasize the utility of these models. The family is a complex unit, the study of which is difficult. In view of the considerable range of data available, such as numbers of births (in toto and by age group), time elapsed since marriage, intervals between births, etc., we do not know exactly which to carry further, because of our inadequate knowledge of their relationships.

The purpose of these models is to advance systematic study of these relationship. This is the case, for example, with the relationship between fertility rates of fecund couples and intervals between births. Knowledge of these relationships considerably facilitates the analytical use of intervals between births and makes it more profitable.

The interpretation of results is another difficulty presented by the study of complex data. Experience shows errors of interpretation to be frequent. This is the case, for example, with birth intervals. Many novices misinterpret observed variations in the mean birth interval according to birth order, attributing to the effects of birth order what, in fact, is due to chance variation between families, the mechanism of which may be well grasped through study of models.

There are cases, furthermore, in which the analysis of results and, *a fortiori,* their interpretation, is almost impossible without recourse to models. One good example is the numerical study reported here of the effect of a decline in fecundability on birth intervals. Working with a model enabled us to carry the analysis and interpretation of the Japanese data to some lengths. Lacking a model, we would have been limited to a description of these data or, at best, to a superficial interpretation of them.

Finally, the last application permitted us to determine the conditions for the use of an analytic procedure which is of great interest but has the disadvantage of introducing a bias. The existence of this bias may be admitted *a priori,* but its significance cannot be evaluated without a model.

CHAPTER FOUR

The Duration
of the Nonsusceptible Period
in Estimates
of Natural Fertility*

EDITORS' SUMMARY

In this paper (published in 1964), M. Henry investigates methods of establishing a lower limit for the mean duration of the nonsusceptible period associated with a live birth as a function of age, when it is assumed that fecundability, the duration of the nonsusceptible period, or both may depend on age. The methods are applied to numerical data.

*Originally printed in French as "Mesure du temps mort en fécondité naturelle." *Population* 19, no. 3 (Juin-Juil. 1964): 485-514.

CONTENTS

INTRODUCTION

A pregnant woman cannot conceive again for a certain period, which ends at the later of two events: the resumption of ovulation or the resumption of sexual relations. Thus each conception marks the beginning of a nonsusceptible period, which is one of the three fundamental functions determining natural fertility. [See Chapter Two, pp. 31–32.]

The duration of the nonsusceptible period is increased by delays in either the resumption of sexual relations or the reappearance of ovulation. It may be prolonged for many months following delivery, either by a taboo on sexual relations during lactation, which exists among certain people, or by prolonged breast feeding, which prevents or delays the return of ovulation in a sizeable fraction of women.

For an individual woman, the duration of nonsusceptibility varies according to the outcome of a pregnancy. In the case of an intrauterine death, it ends only a few weeks after the end of

SUMMARY OF NOTATION

x, t Age of woman, time.

$g(t)$ Duration of the nonsusceptible period, including pregnancy, when the nonsusceptible state ends at t.

$g_m(t)$ Lower limit of g.

$V_g(t)$ Variance of g.

$p(t)$ Fecundability at t.

$c(t)$ In the text and Appendix II: mean conception delay when p does not vary with the woman's age; in Appendix I: $c(t)$ is equal to $\dfrac{1}{p(t)}$; but the functional t is suppressed, so we find only c.

$c_M(t)$ Maximum value of c (when g does not vary with t).

i In the text: characteristic interval, i.e. $c + g$, which exists only where p and g do not vary with the woman's age; in Appendix I: sum of $c(t)$ and $g(t)$; in Appendix II: reference interval in absence of intra-uterine deaths. (These distinctions disappear when p and g do not vary with t; i is then at the same time the characteristic and the reference interval).

$\Lambda(t)$ Mean interval straddling age t.

e Difference between the characteristic interval and the mean straddling interval.

$\bar{\imath}$ Arithmetic mean of characteristic interval.

γ Coefficient of variation corresponding to $\bar{\imath}$.

$J(t)$ Mean of the interval between conceptions that ends in $(t, t + dt)$.

$L(t)$ Mean of the interval between conceptions that begins in $(t, t + dt)$.

$Y(t)$ Reference interval, i.e. arithmetic mean of J and L (used as an estimator of $\bar{\imath}$).

V Variance of intervals between births within families.

$f(t)$ Number of conceptions at time t.

$s(t)$ Number of exits from the nonsusceptible period at time t.

$F(t)$ Number of conceptions in the interval $(t - g, t)$.

Generally the functional (t) will be suppressed except when a time other than t is to be denoted.

the pregnancy. If a woman has had a live birth, the duration of the nonsusceptible period may be shortened by the death of the infant during lactation, by breaking the taboo or by inducing the return of ovulation. It is possible, in addition, that the duration of nonsusceptibility varies with the woman's age, and it is probably shorter after the first birth than after later births. On the one hand, medical writers report that lactation amenorrhea is less frequent after the first delivery than after subsequent ones; on the other hand, the mean interval between two successive births increases with birth order, but not in a regular fashion: the increase from interval 1–2 to interval 2–3 is greater than from interval 2–3 to interval 3–4 (if the latter is neither the last nor the second last).

The duration of nonsusceptibility certainly varies from one woman to another, if only because lactation does not prevent ovulation in some women, while in others it suppresses ovulation totally until weaning or even later. These differences between women seem to be the main reason for differences in fertility; it has been observed, in fact, that the interval following an infant death varies a great deal less with the final size of the family than does a normal interval (i.e. one where the first of two children has reached the age of one year). It would not be so if variation among women were due primarily to differences in fecundability.

DIRECT AND INDIRECT MEASURES

To study this important factor in depth, it would be necessary to estimate the duration of the nonsusceptible period, whether directly or indirectly. A direct estimate of the delay in the reappearance of ovulation would not be very difficult to make for a small sample; it would certainly be much more difficult for a random sample of young women after confinement in a developed society, even if the procedure consisted only of daily temperature recordings, because generally it would not be possible to continue observation for a relatively long time. On the other hand, such observations could include only a few cases where lactation was sufficiently prolonged; the data would not be applicable to patterns of natural fertility in historical populations or in certain underdeveloped modern populations.

It would seem that information regarding the resumption of sexual relations could be obtained more easily, since in some countries subjects have not refused to reply to surveys that ask even more indiscreet questions, but one cannot be certain that they always reply truthfully. In addition, it is not possible to separate the estimation of this delay from that of the anovular period, since the *longer* of the two added to the duration of pregnancy determines the duration of the nonsusceptible period.

Consequently, indirect methods may be preferable. For this purpose, we have data that are relatively easy to obtain, i.e. intervals between live births. These may be considered as equivalent to the intervals between conceptions of live-born children, which are the sum of the duration of the nonsusceptible period that follows such a conception and the delay in the conception of a live-born child after the end of the nonsusceptible period.[1]

---

[1] Analogues to the nonsusceptible period are encountered in many other fields. Thus, a machine breakdown marks the beginning of a period during which it cannot break down again; this period is at least as long as the duration of the breakdown, or it may last longer if the repair eliminates the risk of breakdown for a time. Here the period of repair is analogous to pregnancy, and the period without risk of breakdown that may follow the repair is analogous to the anovular period after delivery. Another analogy is illness: the duration of an illness and the subsequent period of total immunity, if it exists. One could also extend the analogy to accidents, to the extent to which the person suffering an accident protects himself for a time against any danger or against a specified danger.

In such situations, the analogue of the nonsusceptible period may be referred to as "dead time." A dead time exists in the sequence of generations whenever there is a minimum age before reproduction can begin. This is the case for most living beings, and there are perhaps none where generations can follow each other without any delay.

In general, a dead time exists whenever the occurrence of an event prevents a similar event from occurring during a certain period, without appreciably modifying later events.

This restriction distinguishes the problem that concerns us from that of queues. Thus, despite the verbal analogy, artistic or literary fertility may resemble physiological fertility less than does the functioning of a telephone line. The idea for a new artistic work can germinate during the realization of an earlier idea and, after a fashion, take its place in the queue. A telephone call to a busy line (conversation equals dead time) must on the other hand be remade.

One should not conclude from these analogies that the problems of estimating dead time are always identical. In the case of natural fertility, the specific nature of the problem springs from the absence of an observable event (at least in the current state of affairs) marking the end of the nonsusceptible period. Analogues exist for illness (the end of immunity), for breakdown (if the risk of all breakdowns does not reappear until some time

(continued on next page)

[Let the mean conception delay, for a susceptible woman be designated as c and the duration of the nonsusceptible period, including pregnancy, by g. Several different methods of estimating g will now be presented and discussed:

(1) The calculation of the difference between the mean interval between births 1 and 2 and the mean interval from marriage to the first birth.

(2) Two methods used by K. Dandekar based on the variance of four intervals for the same woman. Of these methods, the one that yields the lower estimate of g will be presented in detail.

(3) A method, the basis for which is derived in part in the Appendix, that uses data on intervals which begin and end within a defined age period (called interior intervals) and intervals that "straddle" the two limits of this age period. Using this general approach, but varying the assumptions, several modifications of this estimate will be derived. The consecutive assumptions are:

    (a) a homogeneous population, with fundamental functions constant over time and an invariant g.

    (b) a homogeneous group with random variations in g.

    (c) a heterogeneous group where g and p vary between women.

    (d) g and p are functions of age (theoretical derivations are given in Appendix I).

    (e) the effect of intra-uterine mortality (see Appendix II).

Numerical estimates of g based on these assumptions are made for several sets of data.]

INTERVALS BETWEEN BIRTHS COMPARED TO THE INTERVAL FROM MARRIAGE TO THE FIRST BIRTH

The mean delay to the conception of a live-born child following marriage can be estimated from the mean interval between marriage and the first live birth. If one knew that, at least during

---

after the repair), and perhaps also for the division of unicellular creatures. Analogues would exist in art and in literature, if the completion of a product left the artist without inspiration for some months.

Let us note finally that even for similar problems, the solutions may vary. Thus, for example, the study of intervals between successive attacks of the same disease could relate to the duration of immunity only under conditions that are rarely met. Perhaps because the duration of immunity is too long, or because the spread of an infection changes the risk of contagion greatly, we may be a long way from the model of fertility where the risk of conception varies little outside of periods of immunity.

certain ages, this delay is equal to the conception delay that follows a nonsusceptible period, one could estimate the mean postpartum nonsusceptible period by comparing the mean interval between two consecutive births with the mean interval between marriage and the first birth. The total duration of the nonsusceptible period would then be equal to the duration of the postpartum nonsusceptible period plus nine months.

In the absence of conception, fecundability increases, either suddenly or gradually, until about age 20; apparently it then reaches a plateau. It is unknown whether the first delivery produces a change. Survey data on conception delays after discontinuing contraception do not settle this question, because they are not sufficiently precise. It can be taken as probable that, during full maturity, say from about age 20 to about age 30, the fecundability of young married women is not very different from that of women already mothers and, consequently, that the estimate mentioned above provides an approximation for the postpartum nonsusceptible period.

Consider the marriages occurring in Crulai in 1674–1742. For the 81 women who were married at ages 20-29, conceived their first infant after marriage, and delivered at least twice, the mean interval between marriage and the first delivery is 16.2 months, and that between the first and second delivery is 26.5 months. The duration of the first postpartum nonsusceptible period should then be about 10 months, which [assuming nine months of pregnancy], makes the total duration of nonsusceptibility equal to 19 months. The next nonsusceptible period would last about 21-22 months, if the observed lengthening in the mean intervals between births is attributed to an increase in the duration of nonsusceptibility.[2]

Analogous findings were seen in Mesnil-Theribus among women married at ages 20-29 in 1740–1779. (Ganiage [2][3]). Below are mean values for three successive intervals for the 79 women who delivered at least four times.

Interval	Mean No. of Months
0–1	13.65
1–2	21.20
2–3	24.80

[2] This observation referred only to families of five children or more.

[3] The marriages that occurred after 1779 were eliminated because of the probable beginning of birth limitation.

Assuming constant fecundability, the first nonsusceptible period would last about 16.55 months and the second about 20.15 months.

DANDEKAR'S METHOD

Another method was used by Mrs. K. Dandekar [1, 2];[4] she applied it first to 46 families of Crulai with at least 5 intervals between deliveries, of which the first 4 were normal.[5]

She assumed that fecundability was constant for each couple. Under this assumption, if fecundability is denoted by p the conception delay $c = 1/p$; if, in addition, the mean duration of the nonsusceptible period is equal to g, the characteristic interval $i = g + c$.[6]

Dandekar assumed further that the observed mean interval in each family was equal to its characteristic interval i. She combined this hypothesis with two alternatives relating to the nonsusceptible period: (1) for each woman it has a constant duration, or (2) for each woman it is subject to random fluctuations, such that the probability that the nonsusceptible period terminates is zero until some minimum value, and is subsequently constant. But if this hypothesis were acceptable for normal intervals, which is not certain, it would certainly not be acceptable for all intervals, including those following an infant death, which are definitely shorter. [Dandekar defined the mean delay to conception as following ovulation, i.e. $c_d = \dfrac{1}{p} - 1 = c - 1$. Therefore, $g_d = g + 1$.][7]

---

[4] More recently, the same author has applied this method to data on 44 Indian women and found a mean of 22 months. See Dandekar [2].

[5] An interval is called normal when an infant born at the beginning of the interval (or at least one infant in the case of multiple births) lived for at least one year. Otherwise, the interval is called an interval following a death.

[6] For a population with homogeneous values of p and g, expected values of successive intervals are equal to the characteristic interval only as long as there is no selection due to chance. In a group where almost all women have at least five births but only some have eight or more, the expected value of successive intervals is equal to the characteristic interval for women having had at least five deliveries and is less for those with at least eight deliveries.

[7] The mean conception delay having been calculated following ovulation, the nonsusceptible period includes that part of the menstrual cycle that would have followed the preceding conception and that part of the cycle that preceded the first postpartum ovulation. If one calculates the nonsus-

According to hypothesis (1), the internal variance, V, of intervals between births within families, is equal to $\dfrac{(1-p)}{p^2}$. Hence we have:

$$V = c_d(1 + c_d), \tag{1}$$

which permits c to be estimated.

The value g is then obtained as the difference:

$$g_d = i - c_d. \tag{2}$$

This calculation was made for each of 46 couples. The interpretation of the results may, however, be questioned, since a mean and variance calculated from only 4 intervals are subject to large random fluctuations; given the assumptions the mean of the 46 results (21.4 months) better represents the overall mean.

Hypothesis (2) will not detain us long, because hypothesis (1) yields a lower estimate of the mean value of g. In effect, since random fluctuations in the duration of nonsusceptibility are, presumably, independent of those in the conception delay, the total variance V is equal to the sum of $c_d(1 + c_d)$, the variance of the conception delay, and of V_g, the internal variance of the nonsusceptible period:

$$V = c_d(1 + c_d) + V_g. \tag{3}$$

From Eq. (3) one may derive:

$$c_d = \frac{\sqrt{1 + 4(V - V_g)} - 1}{2} \tag{4}$$

and hence, under hypothesis (2):

$$c_d \leqq \frac{\sqrt{1 + 4V} - 1}{2}. \tag{5}$$

Let us denote by c_M the maximum value of c; c_M is calculated under hypothesis (1) and since

$$g \geqq i - c_M, \tag{6}$$

---

ceptible period in terms of ovulations suppressed or rendered useless (i.e. those that occurred before the resumption of sexual relations), the delay must be increased by a cycle, or approximately one month.

the first hypothesis leads to a minimum estimate of the mean duration of the nonsusceptible period.

Furthermore, the fact that the total time during which women can conceive is limited simultaneously reduces both the mean conception delay and its variance. Since the reduction is relatively more marked for the variance than for the mean, one cannot be very certain in this case, of having a minimum estimate of g. It is therefore somewhat of a disadvantage to start with women who have had at least six deliveries.

ANOTHER METHOD OF ESTIMATING g

HOMOGENEOUS GROUPS

We first consider the simplest case: a homogeneous group with both fecundability and duration of nonsusceptibility constant. We assume, in addition, that the available time for reproduction is sufficiently long for the conception delay to have its expected value.

Consider the continuous case, where the formulas are simpler. Assume that the oscillations in fertility that occur at the beginning of marriage are already damped: for example, we are at the thirtieth birthday of women married before age 25. [See Chapter Two, p. 53.] To simplify further, we will speak of conceptions rather than births. For every woman, her thirtieth birthday falls in an interval between conceptions, if we assume that the time on each side of the thirtieth birthday is sufficiently long to ensure at least one conception. This straddling interval consists of two half-intervals, a left fraction from the previous conception to the thirtieth birthday, and a right fraction from the thirtieth birthday to the next conception (see Chapter Three).

Since the oscillations are damped, fertility is constant at its asymptotic value, i.e. at $\dfrac{1}{g+c}$, with $c = \dfrac{1}{p}$ (since we are in the continuous case). In a period of length g, i.e. from $t - g$ to t, the expected number of conceptions equals $\dfrac{g}{g+c}$. There are therefore $\dfrac{c}{g+c}$ women whose last conception before t is also before $t - g$; for these women the expected interval between this conception and the next is $g + 2c$;[8] for the others this interval is equal to $g + c$.

The expected value, Λ, of the straddling interval is given by:[9]

$$\Lambda = (g + 2c) \cdot \frac{c}{g + c} + (g + c) \cdot \frac{g}{g + c} = g + c + \frac{c^2}{g + c} = i + \frac{c^2}{i},$$

$$(7)$$

_____

[8] We have shown [see Chapter Three, p. 83] that the expected value of the left fraction is equal to that of the right fraction. The left fraction, from the previous conception until t, has a mean duration of $\frac{g}{2}$ for the $\frac{g}{g + c}$ women who conceived in the time $(t - g, t)$. For the $\frac{c}{g + c}$ women who conceived before $t - g$, this interval has a mean duration of $g + u$ where u is the mean interval between the end of the nonsusceptible period and t. Hence the overall interval since the last conception until t [i.e. the left fraction] has a mean duration of

$$\frac{c \cdot (g + u) + g \cdot \frac{g}{2}}{g + c}.$$

The $\frac{c}{g + c}$ women whose last conception occurred before $t - g$ must be susceptible at t. Hence on the assumption of a constant p, the mean duration of time until their next conception is equal to the mean conception delay c. For the $\frac{g}{g + c}$ women who conceived in $(t - g, t)$ the mean time from t until the next conception is $\frac{g}{2} + c$. Hence the overall interval from t to the next conception [right fraction] is equal to $\dfrac{c \cdot c + g\left(\frac{g}{2} + c\right)}{g + c}$ [Translators' correction]. If the left and right fractions are equal,

$$\frac{cg + cu + g^2/2}{g + c} = \frac{c^2 + g^2/2 + gc}{g + c}, \text{ then } u = c$$

and hence $g + u + c = g + 2c$.

_____

[9] The longer an interval is, the greater is its chance of straddling a specified age. Hence, there are relatively more long intervals among straddling intervals than among all intervals.

where i designates the characteristic interval $(g + c)$. Thus we have:

	Women Who Conceived in $t - g, t$	Women Who Conceived before $t - g$	All Women
Expected proportion	$\dfrac{g}{g+c}$	$\dfrac{c}{g+c}$	1
Mean left fraction from last conception to t	$\dfrac{g}{2}$	$g + u = g + c$	$\dfrac{c(g+u) + g\left(\dfrac{g}{2}\right)}{g+c}$
Mean right fraction from t to next conception	$\dfrac{g}{2} + c$	c	$\dfrac{c \cdot c + g \cdot \left(\dfrac{g}{2} + c\right)}{g+c}$
Straddling interval	$g + c$	$g + 2c$	$g + c + \dfrac{c^2}{g+c}$

Putting $\Lambda - i = e$, we obtain:

$$c = \sqrt{ei} \quad \text{and} \quad g = i - \sqrt{ei}. \tag{8}$$

The value of i can be estimated by calculating a weighted mean of straddling and interior intervals [i.e. by putting Eq. (59) of Chapter Three equal to i]. Assume the conditions for applying Eq. (8) have been fulfilled. A hypothetical numerical example with values resembling those of the observations in Crulai would yield:

Characteristic interval, i	28.5
Straddling interval, Λ	30
Difference, e	1.5
Product ei	42.75
Square root	6.54
$g = 28.50 - 6.54$	21.96

In practice, things are not so simple:

(1) Even if g could be considered constant, this could be the case only for its mean value (if only because g varies according to whether the child reaches the age of one year or dies before its first birthday).

(2) Both c and g may vary with the woman's age. This is certainly so in the case of c. As for g, there seems to be a difference between the first interval and the second, but it is still unknown if there are other variations.

Variations in these functions will be considered below.

RANDOM VARIATIONS IN g

We have shown that one has, for a homogeneous group as well as for a heterogeneous group (Chapter Three, Eq. (63)):

$$\Lambda = i(1 + \gamma^2), \tag{9}$$

where i is the mean interval between births and γ the coefficient of variation of this interval. [When g is invariant, Eq. (9) reduces to Eq. (7) since, in the continuous case, the variance of the conception delay is equal to c^2, and therefore $\gamma^2 = \dfrac{c^2}{i^2}$.]

In a homogeneous group one has, in the continuous case:

$$V = i^2 \gamma^2 = c^2 + V_g. \tag{10}$$

Consequently:

$$e = \Lambda - i = i\gamma^2 \tag{11}$$

$$ei = i^2 \gamma^2 = c^2 + V_g \tag{12}$$

$$c = \sqrt{ei - V_g} \leq \sqrt{ei} \tag{13}$$

and therefore:

$$g = i - c \geq i - \sqrt{ei}. \tag{14}$$

HETEROGENEOUS GROUPS

The preceding inequality holds for every couple in a heterogeneous group and consequently:

$$\bar{g} \geq \bar{i} - \overline{\sqrt{ei}}, \tag{15}$$

where $\bar{g}$ and $\bar{i}$ are the arithmetic means of g and i and $\overline{\sqrt{ei}}$ the arithmetic mean of the quantities $\sqrt{ei}$.

But $\overline{\sqrt{ei}}$ is less[10] than $\sqrt{\bar{e}} \sqrt{\bar{i}}$ so that if one has:

---

[10] Let x_0 and y_0 be two specific values respectively of the variables x and y. Then:

$$\sqrt{xy} \approx \sqrt{x_0 y_0} + \left(\frac{x - x_0}{2}\right)\sqrt{\frac{y_0}{x_0}} + \left(\frac{y - y_0}{2}\right)\sqrt{\frac{x_0}{y_0}}$$
$$- \frac{1}{8}\left[\frac{(x - x_0)^4}{\sqrt{x_0}}\sqrt{\frac{y_0}{x_0}} - \frac{(y - y_0)^4}{\sqrt{y_0}}\sqrt{\frac{x_0}{y_0}}\right]^2.$$

If x_0 and y_0 are the respective means, and both sides of the equation are summed over all x and y the first degree terms in $(x - x_0)$ and $(y - y_0)$ are equal to zero. The right hand side is then reduced to $\sqrt{x_0 y_0}$ and a negative term. Hence $\sqrt{xy} < \sqrt{x_0 y_0}$.

$$\bar{g} \geq \bar{\imath} - \sqrt{\overline{e\imath}}, \tag{16}$$

necessarily:

$$\bar{g} \geq \bar{\imath} - \sqrt{\bar{e}}\,\sqrt{\bar{\imath}}. \tag{17}$$

VARIATIONS, WITH AGE, IN FECUNDABILITY AND IN DURATION OF NONSUSCEPTIBILITY

Since at least one of the quantities c and g varies with the woman's age, we must see if it is necessary to modify the above results in order to take this variation into account, and how. We know little about the variations whose effects we wish to study; it is, however, probable that for most of the fecund period, say from about age 20 to about age 35 or 40, the variations in fecundability and in the duration of the nonsusceptible period are approximately linear and the rate of change is sufficiently slow to permit us to ignore second order terms. The derivation of results for this case is given in Appendix I.

In this case, the straddling interval is affected by the characteristics of both the preceding age period and the subsequent age period. It is consequently natural to compare the straddling interval with another interval that is also affected by these characteristics. We will choose a weighted mean of the intervals beginning or ending in a conveniently chosen small age interval. In this case, where the fundamental functions vary with age, we will refer to this weighted mean as the *reference interval* and designate it by Y.[11] Appendix I shows that the age for which Y is calculated depends on the assumptions:

(a) If fecundability alone varies, the comparison involves straddling and reference intervals corresponding to the same age.

(b) If the duration of the nonsusceptible period varies, it is necessary to compare the straddling interval at any age t with the reference interval corresponding to a slightly earlier age, $t + \Delta t$, where Δt is given in Eq. (A53).

(c) If the duration of the nonsusceptible period and the conception delay both increase with age, the necessary modification is in the same direction as in (b), but it has a smaller absolute value.

---

[11] When fecundability and the duration of nonsusceptibility are invariant, the reference interval is equal to the characteristic interval; but when fecundability and duration of nonsusceptibility vary there no longer is a characteristic interval. In the Appendix, a method is developed to use Y in estimating g as a substitute for i in the analogue to Eq. (8).

We will assume that only one of these three cases will occur in a specified age interval.[12]

EFFECTS OF INTRA-UTERINE MORTALITY

We show in Appendix II that there is no appreciable error in the estimated lower limit of the duration of the nonsusceptible period when the calculations are based on intervals between live births or presumed live births (infants privately baptized[13] and baptized) rather than on intervals between conceptions without intervening miscarriages.

EXAMPLE OF CALCULATIONS

Since populations are always heterogeneous, we must pay attention to the phenomenon of selection. For a straddling interval, there is no problem; each family is equally represented since it is represented by one interval and one alone. This would not be the case for the mean reference interval, if the latter were to be calculated as the mean of all intervals that begin or end, say, in the span from six months before to six months after a specified age. The probability that an interval between births begins or ends in this span is equal to the probability of a conception in that year: a probability that is higher for some couples (high fecundability, short duration of nonsusceptibility) than for others.

The correct calculation is to determine a reference interval for each family, and then calculate the mean reference interval for the families studied. The problem is thus to evaluate the reference interval for each couple.

Practically no interval between births is longer than five years, so that all women fertile on both sides of an age group, 25–29 years for example, have at least one birth in this group. The reference interval in the age group 25-29 for the couple considered, when variations in the duration of the nonsusceptible period and the conception delay are assumed to be linear, is equal to the reference interval at 27.5 years.

---

[12] We remark, however, that before age 20 one could very well have a decrease in conception delay, associated with an increase in the duration of the nonsusceptible period.

[13] Since private baptism was performed in case of doubt, i.e. when it was uncertain whether the infant was alive, births presumed alive include some infants that would today be considered stillbirths.

TABLE 1

INTERVALS TO BIRTHS OCCURRING AFTER AGE 25.
THREE VILLAGES OF L'ILE DE FRANCE (WOMEN GIVING BIRTH
BEFORE AGE 25, LAST BIRTH AT AGES 40-49)

Family Number	Intervals in Months						
	Straddling Age 25	Interior	Straddling Age 30	Interior	Straddling Age 35	Interior	Straddling Age 40
1	22	22, 16	17	20, 18	18	20, 18	21
2	23	12, 15, 15	19	30	32	——	55
3	19	35	23	30	19	24, 15	22
4	22	12, 13, 22	12	21, 10, 14	14	12, 22, 17	12
5	18	18, 19	20	23, 22	21	23	21
6	24	32	28	18, 21	19	16, 23	39
7	13	14, 13, 14	13	13, 16, 16	43	——	39
8	22	28, 24	19	26, 11	26	——	40
9	18	21, 19	20	40	39	——	35
10	19	18, 17	24	25	27	——	63
11	31	20	30	20, 22	29	19	23
12	22	22, 24	17	24, 23	24	27	18
13	22	23, 31	32	24	23	27	24
14	13	22, 15	23	——	53	16, 31	27
15	25	30	25	19, 25	39	24	21
16	15	21, 22	36	——	35	38	62
17	23	35	24	24	47	22	66
18	25	32	29	28	30	24	34
19	20	29	69	——	41	——	50

Note: The straddling intervals have been derived from the data from the work of J. Ganiage [2] (pp. 143-146, Table III). For example, the first woman appearing in that table married at age 18 (in completed years), and had successive intervals of length 10, 14, 28, 14, 22, 22, 16, 17, 20, 18, 18, 20, 18 and 21 completed months. It is assumed that all marriages occur half-way between two birthdays, e.g. for this first woman at exactly 18½ years (eighteen months before the twentieth birthday). To -18 months one adds successively the odd numbered intervals in completed months and the even numbered intervals increased by one i.e. 10, 15, 28, 15, 22, 23, 16. . . ., (a convenient procedure for taking account of the fact that an interval x in completed months is equal, on the average, to $x + 0.5$). Thus, one has the series of partial totals -8, 7, 35, 50, 72, etc. The second interval (14 months) is straddling age 20 (month zero), the fifth interval (22 months) is straddling age 25 (month 60).

To compare this reference interval to the straddling interval one may:

— either compare the straddling intervals at 25, 30, and 35 years to the arithmetic means of the reference intervals at 22.5 and 27.5 years, . . . , 32.5 and 37.5 years; or

— compare the reference intervals at 27.5, 32.5, and 37.5 years to the arithmetic means of the straddling intervals at 25 and 30 years, 30 and 35 years, 35 and 40 years.

We have chosen the second procedure because the paucity of observations on women married and mothers before age 20 makes it impossible to calculate the reference interval at 22.5 years. In practice, the reference interval at 27.5 years is the weighted mean of intervals having their beginning, their end, or both, between the woman's twenty-fifth and thirtieth birthdays, the weights for interior intervals being twice those for straddling intervals.

Table 1 shows data relating to 19 women from three villages of l'Oise (Mesnil-Theribus, Marcheroux, Beaumont-les-Nonains) married between 1740 and 1779 and giving birth before age 25. It gives the intervals straddling ages 25, 30, 35, and 40 and the interior intervals for ages 25–29, 30–34, and 35–39, all in elapsed months. The reference interval Y of the first couple at 25–29, [calculated according to Eq. (59) of Chapter Three] is:

$$0.5 + \frac{22 + 2(22) + 2(16) + 17}{6} = 19.7$$

where 0.5 is added since the data are given in elapsed months. The mean reference interval at age 27.5, for all nineteen couples, is equal to:

$$\frac{19.7 + 16.3 + \ldots + 37.3}{19} \ .$$

First Example

For the same villages, from tables similar to that just used, we calculated, for age groups 25-29, 30-34, and 35-39, the straddling intervals at their limits and the reference interval; we then made the same calculations for age groups 27.5–32.4 and 32.5–37.4. The results are given in Tables 2a and 2b.

Table 2(a)
Straddling and Reference Intervals
for Age Groups 25–29, 30–34, and 35–39

Interval	Age								
	25	27.5	30	30	32.5	35	35	37.5	40
Straddling	22.0		26.4	25.9		32.2	30.3		37.7
Reference		23.8			27.2			31.5	
Number of women		28			58			49	

[Note: Two values are given for straddling intervals at certain ages. For example in Table 2(a), for the 28 women included in the 25–29 year age group, the mean length of the interval straddling age 30 was 26.4 months, but for the 58 women in the 30–34 year age group, the mean was 25.9 months.]

TABLE 2(b)

STRADDLING AND REFERENCE INTERVALS

FOR AGE GROUPS 27.5–32.4 AND 32.5–37.4

Interval	Age					
	27.5	30	32.5	32.5	35	37.5
Straddling	24.6		30.2	28.5		33.3
Reference		25.8			28.85	
Number of women		38			49	

Figure 1, which illustrates this table, shows that the change in the mean intervals with age is approximately linear, as was expected. Although the slope is not flat (in five years the increase in the intervals is about four months, that is to say one-seventh to one-sixth of the initial values), it is sufficiently so to disregard the second order terms.

TABLE 3

RESULTS OF THE VARIOUS CALCULATIONS

TO ESTIMATE THE LOWER LIMITS OF g, g_m (1ST SERIES)

(INTERVAL LENGTHS IN MONTHS)

	Age x				
	27.5	30	32.5	35	37.5
$\Lambda\,(x)$	24.5	26.8	29.2	31.5	33.9
$Y\,(x)$	23.6	25.5	27.3	29.1	31.0
e	0.9	1.3	1.9	2.4	2.9
eY	21.24	33.15	51.87	69.84	89.90
$\sqrt{eY}$	4.6	5.8	7.2	8.4	9.5
g_m (1st series)	19.0	19.7	20.1	20.7	21.5

From the regression lines, we obtain the values shown in Table 3[14] for Λ and Y, and, by subtraction, the values of e, obtained by substituting Y for i in Eq. (11). To calculate corresponding lower limits of g, g_m (for a specified age) we use the relation from Eq. (14):

---

[14] Table 3 is a combination of the two small tables appearing on pp. 496 and 497 of the French text.

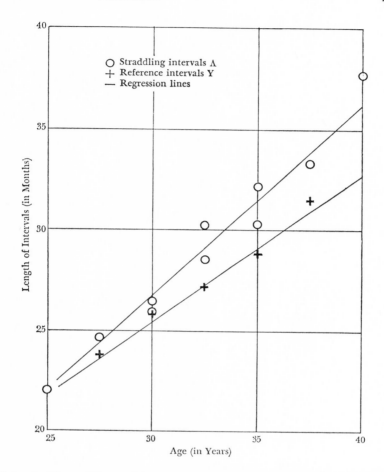

Figure 1. Three villages of l'Ile de France, marriages between 1740 and 1779; length of straddling and reference intervals, by age of woman from Tables 2a and 2b.

$$g_m = Y - \sqrt{eY}. \tag{18}$$

But to take account of possible variations in the duration of the nonsusceptible period, we must also compare Λ at age x with the reference interval corresponding to a lower age, $x - \Delta x$. In this way we will obtain lower values for g_m. A first attempt shows that the estimates decrease by not more than one and one-half months. Since the maximum Δx corresponds to the minimum

TABLE 4

RESULTS OF THE VARIOUS CALCULATIONS
TO ESTIMATE THE LOWER LIMITS OF g, g_m (2ND AND 3RD SERIES)

	Age				
	27.5	30	32.5	35	37.5
g_m (2nd series)	17.5	18	18.5	19	20
Δx	4.8	5.8	6.7	7.4	8.1
ΔY	0.30	0.36	0.41	0.46	0.50
$Y(x - \Delta x) = Y - \Delta Y$	23.3	25.1	26.9	28.6	30.5
$e_2 = \Lambda(x) - Y(x - \Delta x)$	1.2	1.7	2.3	2.9	3.4
$e_2 \cdot Y(x - \Delta x)$	27.96	42.67	61.87	82.94	103.70
$\sqrt{e_2 \cdot Y(x - \Delta x)}$	5.3	6.5	7.9	9.1	10.1
new $g_m{}^*$ (3rd series)	18.0	18.6	19.0	19.5	20.4

$^*g_m = Y(x - \Delta x) - \sqrt{e_2 \cdot Y(x - \Delta x)}$

g_m [see Appendix I, Eq. (A53) and (A54)], we calculate the maximum Δx by the formula:

$$\text{Max. } \Delta x = \frac{Y(Y - g_m)}{2Y - g_m} \qquad (19)$$

using the values for g_m (second series) shown in Table 4.[15]

Y increases by 7.4 months in 10 years, and consequently by 0.74 months per year. If both variables are measured in months, $\Delta Y = \dfrac{0.74 \, \Delta x}{12}$. Δx and ΔY as well as $Y(x - \Delta x) = Y(x) - \Delta Y$ are shown in Table 4 together with the subsequent calculations. When the values $Y(x - \Delta x)$ are subtracted from Λ, we obtain a new series of differences e_2, of products $e_2 \, Y(x - \Delta x)$, of square roots of these products, and of values g_m (see Table 4).

The two series of lower limits for the duration of nonsusceptibility are approximately parallel, with a difference of a little more than one month. But one part of these figures should be rejected. The first series was obtained by supposing the nonsusceptible period to be invariant. If this hypothesis is maintained, only the highest value of the series can be retained without a contradiction; therefore the nonsusceptible period would last at least 21.5 months. The second series corresponds to the other extreme hypothesis: only the duration of the nonsusceptible period varies; in this case it should vary as much as the reference interval. Thus

---

[15] Table 4 is the result of the combination of the three tables appearing on page 498 of the French text.

TABLE 5

SERIES OF LOWER LIMITS OF g WHEN ONLY
THE DURATION OF NONSUSCEPTIBILITY VARIES

	Age				
	27.5	30	32.5	35	37.5
g_m	18.0	19.9	21.7	23.5	25.4

one obtains a new series of lower limits for g, starting with the lowest value, 18.0, at age 27.5 and adding to it the increase in $Y(x - \Delta x)$. The results (fourth series) are as in Table 5.

Figure 2 suggests that one could derive still lower estimates of g_m, except for very young ages, by adopting an intermediate hypothesis, that the increase in the duration of the nonsusceptible period is parallel to that in the first two sets of lower limits that were calculated. The reference interval increases by 7.4 months in 10 years; g_m increases by about 2.5 months in one series, by 2.4 in the other, that is to say by about one-third as much as the increase in the reference interval. Calculating a new value for Δx, we obtain 1.4 months.[16] The value of ΔY corresponding to this value of Δx, is $\Delta Y = 0.09$, which we round to 0.1. Therefore we have to decrease the values of Y in Table 3 by 0.1 and to increase those of e by 0.1 (which gives us e_3). Table 6 shows the calculation of these new estimates of g_m (fifth series).

TABLE 6

CALCULATION OF THE 5TH SERIES OF g_m

	Age				
	27.5	30	32.5	35	37.5
$Y(x - \Delta x)$	23.5	25.4	27.2	29.0	30.9
e_3	1.0	1.4	2.0	2.5	3.0
$\sqrt{e_3\, Y(x - \Delta x)}$	4.8	6.0	7.4	8.5	9.6
g_m	18.7	19.4	19.8	20.5	21.3

From these results, we conclude that the lower limit of the duration of the nonsusceptible period has a mean of about twenty months, in the age interval 27.5–37.5 years.

---

[16] With $c' = 2g'$, $i = 27$, $c = 7.5$, $g - 19.5$, we have from Eq. (A53),
$$\Delta x = \frac{27 \times 7.5 \times 19.5}{2(27^2 + 2 \times 7.5 \times 27 - 7.5^2) + (27^2 - 7.5^2)} = \frac{3948}{2829} = 1.4$$
[where Δx is equal to $- \Delta t$ —L.H.].

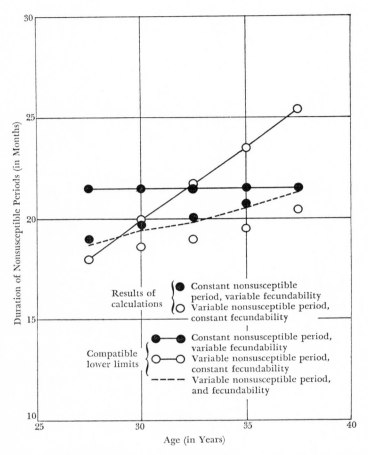

Figure 2. Three villages of l'Ile de France: estimated lower limits of the non-susceptible period, by age of woman.

SECOND EXAMPLE

At Crulai[17] (marriages of 1674–1742) the values of the straddling and reference intervals are shown in Table 7.

Figure 3, showing these values, suggests that we should replace the two values of Λ at age 30 by their mean (30.1), and leave the others unchanged: one can, on the other hand, compare the mean at 30 years, 30.1 months to the mean (28.6 months) of the values of Y at 27.5 and at 32.5 years of age.

---

[17] This concerns the same groups as in the article already cited.

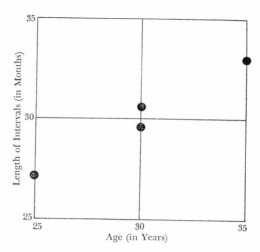

Figure 3. Crulai, marriages from 1673–1742: length of straddling intervals, by age of woman.

TABLE 7
VALUES OF THE STRADDLING AND REFERENCE INTERVALS AT CRULAI

	Age					
	25	27.5	30	30	32.5	35
Straddling	27.2		30.6	29.6		33.0
Reference		27.1			30.1	
Number of women		51			65	

The calculation of g_m without a shift in x is then as in Table 8.

TABLE 8
ESTIMATES OF g_m WITHOUT SHIFT ΔY FOR THE DATA OF CRULAI

	Age		
	27.5	30	32.5
Λ	28.65	30.1	31.55
Y	27.1	28.6	30.1
e	1.55	1.5	1.45
$\sqrt{eY}$	6.5	6.55	6.6
g_m	20.6	21.95	23.5

TABLE 9

ESTIMATES OF g_m INCLUDING ΔY FOR CRULAI

	Age		
	27.5	30	32.5
$Y - \Delta Y$	26.7	28.2	29.7
e	1.95	1.90	1.85
$\sqrt{e(Y - \Delta Y)}$	7.2	7.3	7.4
g_m	19.5	20.9	22.3

Now let us introduce the adjustment. With 19, 20.5, and 22 as approximate values for g_m, one obtains for Δx, 6.2, 6.3 and 6.4 months respectively. Hence we can estimate for [ΔY —L.H.] a rounded adjustment of 0.4 months at the three ages. The calculations for this procedure are shown in Table 9.

But since the second series is calculated on the assumption that only the duration of nonsusceptibility increases, it is necessary, as before, to try to replace it by a series calculated by adding to the lowest value, 19.5, the increase in Y from 27.5 to 30 years, and from 27.5 to 32.5 years. This gives for ages 27.5, 30, and 32.5 respectively, values of g_m equal to 19.5, 21.0, and 22.5 months.

In contrast to the earlier example, this series gives values scarcely in excess of those in the first series.

SUMMARY AND CONCLUSION

The two examples lead to analogous conclusions: (a) Nonsusceptible periods are long since they must exceed the rather high values found for the lower limits; (b) The lower limits increase with the woman's age.

Let us examine these two points in order.

(a) Toward age 30, the lower limit of the duration of nonsusceptibility is about twenty months, a little lower at Mesnil-Théribus, a little higher in Crulai. Since there is about one month between two successive menstrual cycles, we must subtract one month from the preceding result so as to keep only what belongs to pregnancy; thus one obtains the value 19 months.

On the other hand, premature infant death reduces the nonsusceptible period by five months on the average at Mesnil-Théribus, and by almost nine months in Crulai. The infant mortality rates are between one-fifth and one-fourth. In the absence of infant death, the length of the nonsusceptible period would then be increased by one or two months above its overall value.

Thus we return to a minimum of at least 20 months for women at age 30. This means that the mean duration of postpartum non-susceptibility was at least 11 months for women of this age, as a result of either the absence of sexual relations or the absence of ovulation.

It is known, from dictionaries of "cases of conscience," from the catechism for married people by R. P. Feline, from a citation of Restif de la Bretonne as quoted by J. Houdaille [1], that there was at least a tendency to abstain from sexual relations during lactation, particularly when a woman was nursing a child not her own. There was certainly no strict rule, perhaps not even a custom, and it probably was followed relatively little because of the reservations of the Church and the difficulty of prolonged continence in a state of strict monogamy.[18] Accordingly, non-susceptibility would follow primarily from the absence of ovulation for at least an appreciable fraction of women during lactation. That this nonsusceptibility exists was always known by the folk, but since exceptions were not uncommon, some authors considered it a baseless popular belief.

Now, the absence of ovulation during at least a part of lactation can be taken as a fact, not as an absolute rule but in terms of a statistical law. The frequent amenorrhea during all or part of the period of lactation is most often associated with an absence of ovulation,[19] according to biopsies and temperature curves during postpartum amenorrhea.

At about age 30, the lower limit of the duration of the non-susceptible period differs relatively little from the estimate for the second nonsusceptible period,[20] on the assumption that fecundability remains at the same level as at the beginning of marriage. This indicates that if the first delivery causes a discontinuity in the level of fecundability, it would tend to be in the direction of an increase.

(b) The estimated lower limits of the duration of the nonsusceptible period increase with the woman's age. The difference between the nonsusceptible period and its lower limit result from

---

[18] In order to avoid opportunity for temptation to adultery, the Church is not in favor of abstention during lactation without serious reason.

[19] [Except in cases where the first ovulation leads to a conception, amenorrhea is always associated with anovulation.]

[20] That following the second conception of a live-born child.

its variance. *A priori,* it is tempting to suppose that the latter represents an almost constant fraction of the variance of the intervals between births; on this hypothesis, the variation in the lower limit of the duration of the nonsusceptible period indicates a parallel variation in the duration of the nonsusceptible period itself.

Available observations do not permit verification of a continuous increase in the duration of nonsusceptibility with age; those from Mesnil-Théribus allow us, at least, to assume that the duration of the nonsusceptible period is greater at age 37.5 than at age 27.5. If this were not the case, the nonsusceptible period at age 27.5 would in fact last longer than 21.5 months. Since, at this age, the reference interval adjusted for the effects of intra-uterine mortality is about 21.5 months, the nonsusceptible period must be shorter than 21.5 months. Therefore there is necessarily an increase in the duration of the nonsusceptible period between ages 27.5 and 37.5, but the increase is not necessarily continuous.

Since lactation amenorrhea is more common after the second delivery than after the first, the nonsusceptible period associated with the second birth could be longer than that associated with the first. Subsequently, it might become stabilized. Its variation with the woman's age would then consist of an increase at a diminishing rate, corresponding to the decreasing frequency of first births as age increases.

In addition, if the duration of nonsusceptibility were stabilized, its variance should decrease greatly with increasing age, because it would approach its lower limits more closely.

In the historical period, it is likely that every woman would have tried to nurse each of her children for the same time, considered optimal at that period. To fix our ideas, suppose that the desired optimum were 15 months, and, for simplicity, that suppression of ovulation never continued after weaning.[21] For some women the nonsusceptible period would last 15 months, except for cessation of lactation because of infant deaths, disease, or accident, or for the premature reappearance of ovulation. For others the nonsusceptible period is normally, say, 14 months, with the same exceptions. One would then expect that a decreased variance of the duration of the nonsusceptible period would be accompanied by an increase in its mean, since for each one of the

---

[21] In reality, the first few cycles have a greater chance than average of being anovular. But this does not affect the reasoning.

categories of women described, the mean will tend to approach the maximum. For the nonsusceptible period to be constant with increasing age, it would be necessary that the maximum durations of nonsusceptibility and the consequent inhibition of ovulation should decrease with increasing age, so as to compensate exactly for the trend in the opposite direction produced by the decreased dispersion.[22]

Under these conditions, the hypothesis of a continuously increasing duration of the nonsusceptible period with increasing age (but not necessarily at a constant rate), appears to be the most plausible.

In view of the data available, one cannot go further without recourse to other sources, especially of medical origin. If it were known, for example, that the durations of lactation amenhorrea for the same woman show little variation, and that temporary pathological postpartum sterility is rare,[23] we would have an idea of the dispersion in the duration of nonsusceptibility and hence of its true value.

If the difficulties resulting from the dispersion in the duration of nonsusceptibility cannot be surmounted, one could attempt to compare the interval from marriage to first birth with intervals between births, while eliminating the discontinuity which may be due to the first delivery. For this, it would be necessary to study the interval to the first birth among remarried widows, with due attention to the effects of the selection associated with remarriage (the chances of remarrying are not independent of the number of children and hence of fecundity).

It would be necessary, at the same time, to be able to allow for the effects of age on the conception delay. Hence this subject would also need further study. Moreover this would be in order to confirm the increase in conception delay with age after age 20–22, rather than to investigate, without previous observations, what variations occur in fertility with age. Such investigations would also increase the available data, which are, at present, very scanty.

With more data, one could undoubtedly investigate possible differences in the duration of the nonsusceptible period in different populations. This is important, because there are, very

---

[22] We exclude the hypothesis of a decrease in the duration of nonsusceptibility because it entails a series of variations in opposite directions: increase, decrease, increase, which appears very unlikely.

[23] Such episodes would greatly increase the variation in the duration of nonsusceptibility.

probably, differences in natural fertility between populations. At present, we do not know what factors determine such differences. We must not, however, be deceived about the difficulties of such observations in the absence of complete birth registration.

Appendix 1

VARIATIONS IN p AND IN g

In this section we will study how variations with age in p and in g affect the relations between straddling intervals and other intervals. Assume that p and g are linear functions of time during a period of at least five years and that their slopes are sufficiently flat to permit one to ignore the squares or the products of the derivatives p' and g'. [If a variable W is a linear function of age (x) so that $W(x) = a + bx$, the derivative $W' = \dfrac{dW(x)}{dx}$ $= b$, i.e. to the slope. If the slope is small (at most < 1), $(W')^2$ $= b^2$ is, of course, smaller.]

Our main object is to compare the mean of the interval [between conceptions] that straddles a time t, a long time after marriage, to a mean of intervals defined in such a way that the relation in Eq. (7) will hold. Intervals that straddle t depend on characteristics of the ages on both sides of t. Their distribution is not identical with those of intervals that either begin or end in $(t, t + dt)$. Hence it is necessary to combine the two in some way, as for example by taking their mean. But we cannot assume, *a priori*, that the relation in Eq. (7) will hold for the mean of intervals that begin or end in $(t, t + dt)$. We seek a parameter, a shift in time Δt, determined in such a way that the mean of the interval that straddles t and the mean of the intervals that begin or end in $(t + \Delta t, t + \Delta t + dt)$ are related by Eq. (7). As in the case when p and g are constant over time, the women observed may be divided into two groups (see page 126). Group I consists of women susceptible at t; their most recent conception occurred before $t - g$, where g is the duration of the nonsusceptible period that ends at time t. Group II consists of women who are in a nonsusceptible period at t; their most recent conception occurred in the interval $(t - g, t)$. By assumption, we are dealing with a homogeneous population whose fecundability depends only on time.[24] Hence women conceiving in $(t, t + dt)$ constitute a representative sample of Group I. It follows that the left fraction of the straddling interval of Group I (i.e. the time since their previous conception) is equal, on the average, to $J(t)$, i.e. to the interval that ends in $(t, t + dt)$. For this same Group I the right fraction of the straddling interval (i.e. the interval from t to the next conception) is equal to $c(t)$, i.e. the conception delay starting from t, since these women are all susceptible at t. For Group II the interval from t to the next conception is equal to the sum of about half of the duration of the nonsusceptible period g plus the mean conception delay following a date close to $t + g/2$.

FUNDAMENTAL RELATIONS

Group I consists of $(1 - F)$ women; their straddling interval is equal to $J + L(t - g) - g$;[25] Group II consists of F women with a straddling interval equal to $L(t - \theta)$, where θ is the mean date of conception in the interval $(t - g, t)$.

We then have:

$$\Lambda = (1-F) [J + L(t-g) - g] + FL(t-\theta). \tag{A1}$$

Since J and L have the same derivative, which is equal to Y', the derivative of Y [see remarks following Eq. (A35), (A39), and (A40)], we may write:[26]

$$L(t - g) = L - gY' \tag{A2}$$

$$L(t - \theta) = L - \theta Y' \approx L - \frac{g}{2} Y',^{27} \tag{A3}$$

---

[24] g can depend on time and on the number of previous pregnancies, without modifying this analysis.

[25] The conception delay following t is equal to the duration of the interval that begins in $(t - g, t - g + dt)$ decreased by g [i.e. $L(t - g) = g + c(t)$].

[26] [If

$$L(t) = \alpha + \beta t$$
$$L(t - g) = \alpha + \beta t - \beta g$$
$$= L(t) - gL' \text{ since } L' = \beta.$$

Suppressing the functional notation (t) and putting $L' = Y'$, we have Eq. (A2). This reasoning is used throughout this Appendix.]

[27] We have, in effect:

$$t - \theta = \frac{\displaystyle\int_0^g (t - x) \, f(t - x) \, dx}{\displaystyle\int_0^g f(t - x) \, dx}$$

(continued on next page)

and therefore, since $J + L = 2Y$,

$$\Lambda = 2Y - gY' - g + \left(L + \frac{g}{2} Y' - 2Y + g\right) F. \tag{A4}$$

Let us put:

$$L = Y + \Delta Y \tag{A5}$$

$$F = \frac{g}{Y} + \Delta F. \tag{A6}$$

The term in F in Eq. (A4) becomes (if we ignore products of ΔF with ΔY or Y'):

$$\left(g - Y + \frac{g}{2} Y' + \Delta Y\right)\frac{g}{Y} - (Y - g) \Delta F. \tag{A7}$$

Hence:

$$\Lambda = Y + \frac{(Y - g)^2}{Y} - \left(1 - \frac{g}{2Y}\right)gY' + \frac{g}{Y} \Delta Y - (Y - g) \Delta F. \tag{A8}$$

We wish to put Eq. (A8) in the form:

$$\Lambda(t) = Y(t + \Delta t) + \frac{[Y(t + \Delta t) - g(t + \Delta t)]^2}{Y(t + \Delta t)}, \tag{A9}$$

which is that of Eq. (7). Up to terms of the second order, Eq. (A9) is equal to:

$$Y + Y'\Delta t + \frac{(Y - g)^2 + 2(Y - g)(Y' - g')\Delta t}{Y} \cdot \left(1 - \frac{Y'}{Y}\Delta t\right), \tag{A10}$$

---

with

$$f(t - x) = f - f'x.$$

Therefore:

$$\int_0^g f(t - x)\,dx = fg - f'\frac{g^2}{2}$$

$$\int_0^g xf(t - x)\,dx = f\frac{g^2}{2} - f'\frac{g^3}{3}$$

and

$$\theta = \frac{f\frac{g^2}{2} - f'\frac{g^3}{3}}{fg - f'\frac{g^2}{2}} \approx \frac{g}{2} - \frac{f'g^2}{f\,12}.$$

which may be written, omitting terms in $(\Delta t)^2$, as:

$$Y + \frac{(Y-g)^2}{Y} + \left[Y' + \frac{2(Y-g)(Y'-g')}{Y} - \frac{(Y-g)^2}{Y^2} Y' \right] \Delta t.$$
(A11)

The required result is reached by equating Eq. (A8) with Eq. (A11), i.e. where:

$$\left[Y' + 2(Y-g) \frac{(Y'-g')}{Y} - \frac{(Y-g)^2 Y'}{Y^2} \right] \Delta t =$$

$$- \left(1 - \frac{g}{2Y} \right) gY' + \frac{g}{Y} \Delta Y - (Y-g) \Delta F.$$
(A12)

To calculate the value of Δt that will satisfy (A12), we must relate the various functions and their derivatives to p, g and their derivatives, p' and g'.

CALCULATION OF THE DIFFERENT FUNCTIONS

Since fecundability and the duration of nonsusceptibility are assumed to be linear functions of time, one may write:

$$p(t-x) = p - p'x$$
(A13)

$$g(t-x) = g - g'x.$$
(A14)

By definition, for $g(t-x)$, $t-x$ is the date of emerging from the nonsusceptible period. It is convenient, however, in some cases, also to be able to express g as a function of the date of entry, i.e. $g_1(t-x)$. We have:

$$g_1(t-x) = g[t-x+g_1(t-x)] = g(t-x) + g'g_1(t-x)$$
(A15)

and hence:

$$g_1(t-x) = \frac{g(t-x)}{1-g'} \approx (1+g')\, g(t-x).$$
(A16)

Women who conceive in the course of a time interval of length dt leave the nonsusceptible period over a time interval $(1 + g')dt$, because of the prolongation $g'dt$ of the nonsusceptible period in the interval dt. We then have:

$$(1 + g')\, s(t-x)\, dx = f[t-x-g(t-x)]\, dx$$
(A17)[28]

---

[28] Eq. (A17) is the translators' correction.

and since

$$f[t - x - g(t - x)] \approx f - (x + g)\, f', \tag{A18}$$

if follows that

$$s(t - x) \approx [f - (x + g)\, f']\, (1 - g') = f - fg' - gf' - xf' = h - xf' \tag{A19}$$

where

$$h = f - fg' - gf'. \tag{A20}$$

Since fertility is equal to the product of fecundability by the proportion susceptible, i.e. by $(1 - F)$, we have:

$$f = p(1 - F) \tag{A21}$$

$$f' = p'(1 - F) - pF', \tag{A22}$$

with

$$F = \int_0^g f(t - \xi)\, d\xi = fg - \frac{f'g^2}{2}, \tag{A23}$$

and

$$F' = f - (1 - g')\, f(t - g) \approx f - (1 - g')\, (f - f'g) \approx fg' + gf'. \tag{A24}$$

Hence:

$$(1 + pg)\, f = \left(1 + f'\frac{g^2}{2}\right) p \tag{A25}$$

$$(1 + pg)\, f' \approx (1 - fg)\, p' - fpg'. \tag{A26}$$

If $c = \dfrac{1}{p}$, $c' = -p'c^2$. Using this relation, and $i = g + c$, we substitute in Eqs. (A23) to (A26) to derive the results (ignoring products of derivatives):[29]

---

[29] [From the definitions of c and i, we have $i = \dfrac{1 + pg}{p}$, and then Eq. (A25) can be written as follows:

$$if = 1 + \frac{f'\, g^2}{2},$$

$$f \approx \frac{1}{i} + \frac{f'\, g^2}{2i}.$$

Ignoring the products of derivatives to calculate f', we replace f by $1/i$ in Eq. (A26). We then have:

$$if' \approx \left(1 - \frac{g}{i}\right)\frac{p'}{p} - \frac{g'}{i}.$$

$$f \approx \frac{1}{i} - (g' + c') \frac{g^2}{2\,i^3} \qquad (A27)$$

$$f' \approx -\frac{g' + c'}{i^2} \qquad (A28)$$

$$F \approx \frac{g}{i} - (g' + c') \left(\frac{g^3}{2\,i^3} - \frac{g^2}{2\,i^2} \right) = \frac{g}{i} + (g' + c') \frac{cg^2}{2\,i^3} \quad (A29)$$

$$F' \approx \frac{g'c - gc'}{i^2} \, . \qquad (A30)$$

Function J. $s(t - x)\, dx$ women are expected to emerge from the nonsusceptible period in $(t - x,\ t - x + dx)$. Among them the proportion who have not yet conceived again by time t is equal to:[30]

$$e^{-px\,+\,p'\,\frac{x^2}{2}} \approx \left(1 + p'\,\frac{x^2}{2} \right) e^{-px}. \qquad (A31)$$

Therefore, the number of women who have not yet conceived again at time t is:

$$s(t - x) \left(1 + p'\,\frac{x^2}{2} \right) e^{-px}\, dx. \qquad (A32)$$

Replacing $\dfrac{p'}{p}$ by $- c'/c$, we obtain:

$$if' \approx -\left(\frac{i - g}{i} \right)\left(\frac{c'}{c} \right) - \frac{g'}{i} \approx -\frac{c'}{i} - \frac{g'}{i} \,,$$

since $i - g = c$.
We finally have:

$$\left. f' \approx -\frac{c' + g'}{i^2} \right].$$

[30] As in all analogous problems (mortality, nuptiality), the exponent of e is negative and equal in absolute value to the integral of the instantaneous risk of the event considered (here conception):

$$\int_{t-x}^{t} p(u)\, du = -\int_{x}^{0} p(t - \xi)\, d\xi = \int_{x}^{0} (p - p'\xi)\, d\xi = px - p'\frac{x^2}{2}.$$

The integral of (A32) overall values of x, is equal to the number in group I, $1 - F = f/p$.[31]

The mean interval between [the emergence from the nonsusceptible state] and t can be obtained from Eqs. (A19) and (A32), as:

$$\left(\int_0^\infty x(h - xf')\left(1 + p'\,\frac{x^2}{2} \right) e^{-px}\,dx \right) \div \frac{f}{p}, \qquad (A33)$$

which gives:

$$\frac{1}{p}\left[\frac{h}{f} - \frac{2f'}{fp} + \frac{3p'}{p^2} \right] = \frac{1}{p}\left[1 - \frac{F'}{f} - \frac{2f'}{fp} + \frac{3p'}{p^2} \right]$$

$$\approx c\left[1 + (g' + c')\frac{c}{i} - 2c' \right]. \qquad (A34)$$

To derive J, it is still necessary to add the mean duration of the nonsusceptible period that ends at $t - x$; the duration of this period, written $g - g'x$, has a mean value equal to the sum of g plus the product of the result in Eq. (A34) multiplied by $-g'$. Thus, as an approximation up to the second order:

$$J \approx g + (1 - g')\,c\left[1 + (g' + c')\frac{c}{i} - 2c' \right]$$

and

$$J \approx i + c\left[(g' + c')\frac{c}{i} - 2c' \right] - cg' = i - \frac{(2i - c)\,cc'}{i} - \frac{cgg'}{i}.$$

$$(A35)$$

---

[31] Moreover, one can verify this result. One has, in effect from Eqs. (A19) (A20) and (A32):

$$\int_0^\infty (h - xf')\left(1 + p'\,\frac{x^2}{2} \right) e^{-px}dx \approx \frac{h}{p} - \frac{f'}{p^2} + \frac{fp'}{p^3}.$$

Since $f/p = 1 - F$ and h may be written as $f - F'$, the foregoing integral is equal to:

$$1 - F - \frac{F'}{p} - \frac{f'}{p^2} + \frac{fp'}{p^3}.$$

But since, following (A22):

$$\frac{f'}{p^2} = \frac{p'}{p^2}(1 - F) - \frac{F'}{p} = \frac{fp'}{p^3} - \frac{F'}{p}$$

the terms other than $1 - F$ disappear.

The derivative of J is, up to the second order, equal to $c' + g'$, the derivative of i.

Function L. This function is the sum of $g_1(t)$ and the conception delay following $t + g_1(t)$. The conception delay following any date taken as the origin is equal to:

$$\int_0^\infty \xi \, p(\xi) \, e^{-\xi p_0 + \frac{\xi^2}{2}} \, p' \, d\xi \approx$$

$$\int_0^\infty \xi \, [p_0 + p'\xi] \left[1 - p' \, \frac{\xi^2}{2} \right] e^{-\xi p_0} \, d\xi \approx \frac{1}{p_0} - \frac{p'}{p^3{}_0} \quad \text{(A36)}$$

where p_0 is the value of p at the new origin.

Let us now replace p_0 by its value $p(t + g_1)$ as:

$$p_0 = p(t + g_1) \approx p + p'g_1 \approx p + p'g. \quad \text{(A37)}$$

It follows that:

$$\frac{1}{p_0} - \frac{p'}{p_0{}^3} \approx \frac{1}{p}\left(1 - \frac{p'}{p} \, g \right) - \frac{p'}{p^3} = c + ic' \quad \text{(A38)}$$

and using Eq. (A15),

$$L \approx g_1 + c + ic' = g + gg' + c + ic' = i + ic' + gg'.$$
$$\text{(A39)}$$

The derivative of L, like that of J, is equal to $c' + g'$ up to terms of the second order.

Function Y. By definition, $Y = \dfrac{J + L}{2}$ and consequently, from Eqs. (A35) and (A39),

$$Y \approx i + \frac{(i - c)^2}{2i} \, c' + \frac{(i - c)^2}{2i} \, g'. \quad \text{(A40)}$$

The derivative Y' is equal to $c' + g'$, up to terms of the second order.

Calculation of ΔY. From the definition in Eq. (A5) of ΔY (i.e. $\Delta Y = L - Y$) and Eqs. (A39) and (A40):

$$\Delta Y = \frac{i^2 + 2ic - c^2}{2i} \, c' + \frac{i^2 - c^2}{2i} \, g'. \quad \text{(A41)}$$

Calculation of ΔF. From the definition in Eq. (A6), $\Delta F = F - g/Y.$ $\left[\text{ Since } g/Y \text{ may be expressed as } \dfrac{g}{Y} = \dfrac{g}{i\left\{1 + \dfrac{Y-i}{i}\right\}} \approx \dfrac{g}{i}\left\{1 - \dfrac{Y-i}{i}\right\}\right]$, we may put:

$$\Delta F = F - \frac{g}{i}\left(1 - \frac{Y-i}{i}\right) = F - \frac{g}{i} + g\frac{Y-i}{i^2}, \qquad (A42)$$

and replacing F, Y, and g by their expressions as functions of i and c, in Eqs. (A29) and (A40):

$$\Delta F = \left[\frac{c(i-c)^2}{2i^3} + \frac{(i-c)^3}{2i^3}\right](c' + g') = \frac{i(i-c)^2}{2i^3}c' + \frac{i(i-c)^2}{2i^3}g'. \qquad (A43)$$

Calculation of Δt. On substituting the expressions obtained in Eqs. (A41) and (A43) as well as the result $Y' = c' + g'$ in Eq. (A12), and putting $\dfrac{1}{Y} = \dfrac{1}{i}$, we obtain an expression:

$$(Cc' + Dg')\Delta t = Ac' + Bg' \qquad (A44)$$

where A and B are functions only of i and c.

Calculation of A, the Coefficient of c'. One obtains up to terms of the second order:

$$A = -g\left(1 - \frac{g}{2i}\right) + \frac{g}{i} \cdot \frac{(i^2 + 2ic - c^2)}{2i} - \frac{i(i-g)(i-c)^2}{2i^3}. \qquad (A45)$$

The sum of the first and the third terms is equal to:

$$-\frac{i^2(i-c)(i+c) + ic(i-c)^2}{2i^3} = -\frac{i-c}{i} \cdot \frac{(i^2 + 2ic - c^2)}{2i}, \qquad (A46)$$

that is to say, to the opposite of the second term. We therefore have $A = 0$.

Calculation of B, the Coefficient of g'. Still up to terms of the second order, one writes:

$$B = -g\left(1 - \frac{g}{2i}\right) + \frac{g}{i}\left(\frac{i^2 - c^2}{2i}\right) - \frac{i(i-g)(i-c)^2}{2i^3}. \tag{A47}$$

The first and the third terms are the same as in A. One therefore has:

$$B = \frac{g[(i^2 - c^2) - (i^2 + 2ci - c^2)]}{2i^2} = -\frac{gc}{i}. \tag{A48}$$

Coefficient of Δt. This is of the form $Cc' + Dg'$ with:

$$C = 1 + 2\frac{(Y-g)}{Y} - \frac{(Y-g)^2}{Y^2} = \frac{(2Y-g)^2 - 2(Y-g)^2}{Y^2} \tag{A49}$$

$$D = 1 - \frac{(Y-g)^2}{Y^2} = \frac{Y^2 - (Y-g)^2}{Y^2} = \frac{g(2Y-g)}{Y^2}, \tag{A50}$$

from which, up to terms of the second order:

$$C = \frac{(i+c)^2 - 2c^2}{i^2} = \frac{i^2 + 2ic - c^2}{i^2}, \tag{A51}$$

$$D = \frac{(i-c)(i+c)}{i^2} = \frac{i^2 - c^2}{i^2}. \tag{A52}$$

We then have:

$$\Delta t = \frac{-gcig'}{(i^2 + 2ic - c^2)c' + (i^2 - c^2)g'}. \tag{A53}$$

At the ages we are considering, c' and g' are either 0 or positive. If c' and g' are 0, Δt is undefined, and all the functions studied are reduced to constants. If g' is 0 and c' is positive, $[\Delta t]$ is 0. If both g' and c' are positive, Δt is negative and its absolute value is below the maximum that it would reach if $c' = 0$, i.e.

$$\text{Max} \, |\Delta t| = \frac{ci}{i+c},$$

which is estimated as

$$\widehat{\text{max}} \, |\Delta t| = \frac{cY}{Y+c}, \tag{A54}$$

since in practice it is Y and not i that is known. $\frac{cY}{Y+c}$ increases with c; but for a fixed value of Y, c cannot exceed $Y - g_m$, where

g_m is the lower limit of g. In the numerical examples considered in the text, this limit is about 18 months when Y is about 24 months; the absolute value of Δt is then less than 0.4 years.

Appendix 2

EFFECT OF INTRA-UTERINE MORTALITY

The best data available to date have been derived by the reconstruction of families from old vital statistics. Observed intervals are intervals between births presumed alive and not intervals between conceptions. We must see what effect the use of such data has on the theory derived for intervals between conceptions.

In a homogeneous group, the quantity $\sqrt{ei}$, which we substract from the reference interval i, in order to obtain a lower limit for g by Eq. (8), is equal to the standard deviation of the interval between conceptions. When we replace conceptions by births presumed alive, the reference interval is modified and the standard deviation becomes that of the interval between births.

Let g_2 and g_1 be the duration of nonsusceptibility corresponding, respectively, to a live birth and to an intra-uterine death and let v be the probability that a conception ends in a live birth. In the absence of intra-uterine death, the reference interval would be equal to $i = g_2 + c$; the mean interval between births presumed alive is (Chapter Three, Eq. (32) with a change in notation) equal to:

$$Y = \frac{g + c}{v}, \qquad \text{with } g = vg_2 + (1 - v) g_1. \qquad \text{(A55)}$$

Y from Eq. (A55) is greater than i as just defined by:

$$\frac{1 - v}{v} g_1 + \frac{c}{v} - c = \frac{1 - v}{v} i_1, \qquad \text{(A56)}$$

where $i_1 = g_1 + c$, is the reference interval that begins at a conception ending in an intra-uterine death.

The mean interval between births presumed alive is v times an interval i, $v(1 - v)$ times the sum of an interval i and an interval i_1, $v(1 - v)^2$ times the sum of an interval i and of two intervals i_1 and so on. In the same way, the second non-central moment m is replaced by:

$$vm + v(1-v)\,[m + 2ii_1 + m_1] + v(1-v)^2\,[m + 4ii_1 + 4m_1] + \ldots$$
$$+ v(1-v)^k\,[m + 2kii_1 + k^2\,m_1] + \ldots \qquad (A57)$$

where m_1 is the second non-central moment of intervals i_1. The coefficient of $2ii_1$ in Eq. (A57) is equal to:

$$v(1-v) + \ldots + kv(1-v)^k + \ldots = v(1-v)\,[1 + 2\,(1-v) + \ldots$$
$$+ k(1-v)^{k-1} + \ldots] = v(1-v)\,\frac{d}{d(1-v)}\left[\frac{1}{v}\right] = \frac{1-v}{v}\,.$$
$$(A58)$$

The coefficient of m_1 in Eq. (A57) is equal to:

$$v(1-v)\,[1 + 4(1-v) + \ldots + k^2\,(1-v)^{k-1} + \ldots] = v(1-v)$$
$$[1 + 2(1-v) + \ldots + k(1-v)^{k-1} + \ldots + 2(1-v) + \ldots$$
$$+ k(k-1)\,(1-v)^{k-1} + \ldots] = v(1-v)\,\frac{d}{d(1-v)}\left[\frac{1}{v}\right] + v(1-v)^2$$
$$\frac{d^2}{d(1-v)^2}\left[\frac{1}{v}\right] = \frac{1-v}{v} + \frac{2(1-v)^2}{v^2}\,. \qquad (A59)$$

The non-central second moment is therefore:

$$m + \frac{2(1-v)}{v}\,ii_1 + \left[\frac{1-v}{v} + \frac{2(1-v)^2}{v^2}\right]m_1. \qquad (A60)$$

To obtain the variance we must subtract:

$$\left(i + \frac{1-v}{v}\,i_1 \right)^2, \qquad (A61)$$

that is to say:

$$i^2 + 2\,\frac{1-v}{v}\,ii_1 + \frac{(1-v)^2}{v^2}\,i_1^2. \qquad (A62)[32]$$

But we have:

$$m = i^2 + V \qquad (A63)$$

and

$$m_1 = i_1^2 + V_1 \qquad (A64)$$

where V and V_1 are the variances of the intervals in the two cases considered.

---

[32] Eq. (A62) is the translators' correction.

The variance is then:

$$V + \left[\frac{1-v}{v} + 2\frac{(1-v)^2}{v^2} \right] V_1 + \left[\frac{1-v}{v} + \frac{(1-v)^2}{v^2} \right] i_1{}^2 \tag{A65}$$

or, neglecting second order terms:

$$V + \frac{1-v}{v} V_1 + \frac{1-v}{v} i_1{}^2. \tag{A66}$$

We conclude from Eq. (A56) that the expected value of the observed reference interval (between births presumed alive) Y, is greater than i by about $\frac{1-v}{v} i_1$. On the other hand, $\sqrt{eY}$ which is expected to be equal to the standard deviation of these intervals is approximately equal to the square root of Eq. (A66). Let us attempt to estimate the magnitude of the quantities involved.

Since we are concerned with a correction factor, we can apply these formulas to a heterogeneous group, using means of the quantities considered. For a conception delay of six months, V is about 36; v is probably about 75 percent and i_1 about ten months (three to four months of nonsusceptibility and six months of conception delay). Finally, we may put V_1 equal to V; in effect, we estimate a minimal value for the duration of nonsusceptibility by assuming zero variance. V then includes only the variance of the conception delay which is also included in V_1. V_1 includes, in addition, the variance of the duration of gestation, which may be neglected, in view of the approximations involved in this calculation.

Instead of $V = 36$ one then has, for the value of Eq. (A66):

$$\frac{36}{0.75} + \frac{0.25}{0.75} \times 100 = 48 + 33 = 81.$$

Instead of subtracting six months from the reference interval, therefore, one subtracts nine months, i.e. three months too many. But, as already mentioned, the reference interval Y is inflated by $\frac{1-v}{v} i_1$, which is also about three months, approximately the same value as the excess subtracted when $\sqrt{eY}$ is subtracted.

We may therefore ignore the errors resulting from the use of intervals between births presumed alive as a substitute for intervals between conceptions of infants born alive without intervening intra-uterine mortality.

CHAPTER FIVE

Intra-Uterine Mortality and Fecundability*

EDITORS' SUMMARY

A great deal of attention has been paid in the literature to the distribution of intervals from marriage until the first live birth. Most data from apparently noncontracepting couples do not agree with models that assume: (a) that fecundability is constant for each woman, (b) that this function has the same value for all women, and (c) that pregnancy wastage may be ignored. In this chapter (published in 1964) M. Henry explores models that relax assumptions (b) and (c) above. He postulates several different combinations of distributions of fecundability, of the incidence of pregnancy wastage and of two constant values of the duration of the nonsusceptible periods following fetal death. He compares values obtained for specified indices from empirical data with the same indices calculated from hypothetical data based on these models.

*Originally printed in French as "Mortalité intra-utérine et fécondabilité."
Population 19, no. 5 (Oct.-Déc. 1964): 899-940.

CONTENTS

INTRODUCTION

Recent reports indicate that spontaneous intra-uterine mortality is higher than was previously believed (French and Bierman [1]). Hence, increased attention has been drawn to this factor in fertility to which we perhaps have not given the importance it deserves. In this article, we propose to examine the effect that high

SUMMARY OF NOTATION

V conceptions	Conceptions that end in a live birth.
A conceptions	Conceptions that end in a spontaneous abortion.
p	Fecundability.
$h(p)$	P.d.f. of p.
g	Duration of the nonsusceptible period.
v	Proportion of conceptions that terminate in a live birth.
$h(v)$	P.d.f. of v.
n	Number of the month of exposure.
k	Number of suppressed cycles associated with an intra-uterine death.
$V(n)$	Number of first V conceptions occurring in month n of marriage.
W	Number of women observed.
q_n	Conditional fertility rate at nth month, i.e. $q_n = \dfrac{V(n)}{1 - \sum\limits_{m=1}^{n-1} V(m)}$
r_n	V conception ratio at nth month, i.e. $r_n = \dfrac{V(n)}{V(n-1)}$.

In the Appendices, some of these symbols are used with different meanings. Some are used only in a few cases to facilitate the writing of the mathematical expressions; they are not included here.

$V_k(k = 0, 1, 2, 3 \ldots)$	Number of first V conceptions in any month, which have been preceded by k A conceptions.
n_j	Number of V conceptions in month j, where $n_j = \sum\limits_{k=0}^{\infty} V_k(j)$.
d_j	Number of intra-uterine deaths occurring in month j.
$a_m(m = 0, 1, 2, \ldots)$	Number of first V conceptions occurring at month $j + m$ to women who are susceptible at beginning of month j, where $a_m = vp(1 - p)^m$.

| c_m | Number of conceptions (A and V) independent of v. c is also used as the coefficient of variation of p and v. |
| γ and α | Coefficients characterizing intra-uterine mortality. |

spontaneous intra-uterine mortality can have on estimates of natural fecundability, already so difficult. [A passage recapitulating the fundamental functions has been omitted here.] For simplicity, in what follows, we will designate conceptions that end in a live birth as V conceptions and those that end in a spontaneous abortion or in a stillbirth as A conceptions.

The duration of a pregnancy that follows an A conception is variable and this is probably also the case for the total nonsusceptible period, but it is unknown whether nonsusceptibility lasts much longer than the pregnancy or if it is only a little longer. Potter [3] assumes, in a recent article, that the nonsusceptible period in this case is equal to the duration of pregnancy plus one month. We will take a similar, more convenient, value as the minimum, but we will also see what would occur if the nonsusceptible period were considerably longer than the pregnancy.

If conceptions were easily observable, intra-uterine mortality would not pose problems for the estimation of fecundability. It does pose such problems because the observations we have are primarily on live births.[1] Besides, the difficulties are due not only to intra-uterine mortality. One tries to estimate fecundability at the beginning of marriage by studying first live births, according to the duration of marriage in months. Difficulties arise because of the placement of marriage in the menstrual cycle, variations in the length of the cycles between women and for the same woman, and variations in the duration of pregnancy. Vincent [1] has carefully studied these difficulties.

Here, they will scarcely disturb us; actually, they affect only the results measured from marriage and, consequently, scarcely

---

[1] Since a fraction of pregnancies pass unnoticed because of intra-uterine mortality, some difficulties would remain if observations referred to pregnancies rather than to live births.

affect comparisons between the models to which we refer and the observations. The elements of the models follow.

ELEMENTS OF THE MODELS

We will equate the month with the menstrual cycle, and will assume that the duration of the nonsusceptible period is measured in whole months.[2] Thus, for an intra-uterine death during the second month of pregnancy, we will take two full months as the minimum nonsusceptible period (this value corresponds to that assumed by Potter [3]).

We assume that fecundability (p) and the proportion of V conceptions (v) do not vary with the woman's age or with the duration of marriage, and that the same holds for the probability that the nonsusceptible period has a specified duration g.[3]

Thanks to the observations of French and Bierman at Kauai, we have a precise idea of intra-uterine mortality from the second month of pregnancy onward. In the study in question, the level is 25 percent; but since intra-uterine mortality is lower for young women than on the average, it is also necessary to see what would occur with lower levels.

Nevertheless there remains a difficulty which is serious at first glance. Intra-uterine mortality during the first month of pregnancy (that is, in fact, during the fifteen days following conception) remains poorly known. It is estimated that losses are very high before and during implantation. However, it is doubtful whether an intra-uterine death before implantation has any influence on the woman's organism, and in particular whether it would involve a nonsusceptible period. This is an important

---

[2] As we have defined the duration of the nonsusceptible period, it is the number of cycles suppressed by a conception. Thus it begins at the end of the cycle in which conception occurred. Intra-uterine deaths in the second month of pregnancy, according to the current definition of the duration of pregnancy, are located in the first cycle suppressed by the conception and we assume that there is still a suppressed cycle whether the intra-uterine death occurs at the beginning or at the end of the second month; this convention is commonly adopted, at least implicitly, in calculations in discrete time.

[3] The hypothesis about the constancy of p, at least during one or two years, is very reasonable for women married at ages 20–29. It is less acceptable when an appreciable proportion of women marry at very young ages; we have, however, had to utilize all the available data to reduce the effects of random fluctuations.

TABLE 1

DISTRIBUTION OF INTRA-UTERINE MORTALITY
BY MONTH OF PREGNANCY

Duration of Pregnancy	Number of Intra-Uterine Deaths
0	0
1	46
2	26
3	17
4	4
5	3
6	1
7	1
8	1
9	1
Total	100

point, because an A conception that is not followed by a non-susceptible period has no detectable effect on the data for live births. We will examine this point by introducing a very high intra-uterine mortality rate, up to 50 percent, in the models.

Table 1 gives the distribution assumed for the incidence of intra-uterine deaths by the duration of pregnancy.[4] The distribution is based on the observations made at Kauai, but with rounded values.

[4] For very high intra-uterine mortality, we should have adopted a different distribution, where half the deaths would have occurred during month zero. But the change in the distribution would increase the volume of the calculations much more than does the change from one intra-uterine mortality rate to another with the same distribution; we therefore have reduced, to the extent possible, the use of several distributions. [Furthermore, to adopt this distribution is equivalent to assuming that all marriages occur 15 days before ovulation instead of being regularly distributed between two successive ovulations. It would have been better to utilize a distribution nearer reality, for example, one assuming that marriages occur uniformly throughout a 30-day-month, except for the first day of the menstrual period and the four following days. This distribution is as follows:

Difference between the month of the intra-uterine death and the month of conception (month counted since marriage)	0	1	2	3	4	5	6	7	8	9
Frequency of intra-uterine deaths (total = 100)	7	37	27	16	6	3	1	1	1	1

The use of this new distribution does not modify the results of the article —L.H.]

TABLE 2

DURATION OF THE NONSUSCEPTIBLE PERIOD
IN THE CASE OF AN A CONCEPTION,
BY TWO DIFFERENT VALUES OF k

Duration of Pregnancy	Duration of the Nonsusceptible Period (i.e. Number of Suppressed Cycles)	
	$k = 1$	$k = 3$
0	1	3
1	2	4
2	3	5
3	4	6
4	5	7
5	6	8
6	7	9
7	8	10
8	9	11
9	10	12

As already indicated, we assume that the duration of the non-susceptible period is equal to an integral number of months. We have adopted the following simple rule: if an intra-uterine death occurs during the nth month of pregnancy, the nonsusceptible period lasts until the end of month $n + k$, k being equal to or greater than one. The woman becomes susceptible again in month $n + k + 1$. In fact, we have only worked with two values of k, $k = 1$ and $k = 3$. Accordingly, the nonsusceptible period for each duration of pregnancy at the moment of the intra-uterine death is as in Table 2.

INDICES USED

Vincent made considerable use of the conditional *monthly fertility rate,* or the number of live births of order 1, per 1,000 women who have still not delivered their first child. We will also use this index, which, in our models, becomes the number of first V conceptions per 1,000 women who have not yet had a first V conception.[5] Gini, several decades ago, used another index: the ratio of first live births in a given month to those of the

---

[5] In the model, all couples are able to procreate and when allowed sufficient time, the proportion that, by chance, will still not have any births, is negligible.

preceding month.[6] In our models, it becomes the ratio of the number of V conceptions of order 1 at any month to the number during the preceding month.

[Let W be the number of women observed and let $V(n)$ be the number of first V conceptions occurring in month n of marriage. Then the fertility rate of Vincent is equal to:

$$q_n = \frac{V(n)}{W - \sum\limits_{m=1}^{n-1} V(m)}, \tag{1}$$

and the V conception ratio is equal to:

$$r_n = \frac{V(n)}{V(n-1)}. \tag{2}$$

When convenient, we will suppress the subscript and refer to the indices q, r, and the ratio of the indices: $\dfrac{1-r}{q}$.]

This selection of indices is motivated by the following considerations. The influence of intra-uterine mortality on the fertility rate (q) is immediately apparent in month 1, since the number of V conceptions changes with intra-uterine mortality, while the initial number of women remains the same. This is not necessarily the case for r, the V conception ratio. As long as no woman has yet emerged from the nonsusceptible period following the first conception (V or A), the number of V conceptions of order 1 is equal to v times the total number of conceptions (V and A). If this holds for at least two months, then the first value, at least, of the V conception ratio is independent of intra-uterine mortality. One can then hope to extract some information from the comparison of these two indices, which are unequally affected by intra-uterine mortality.

HOMOGENEOUS GROUPS
AND HETEROGENEOUS GROUPS

A homogeneous group is one in which all couples have the

---

[6] In a homogeneous group, in the absence of intra-uterine mortality, the expected value of this ratio is equal to 1 minus the fecundability; in heterogeneous groups, the relation is less simple (cf. Appendix 4).

same characteristics: fecundability, intra-uterine mortality, and nonsusceptibility.

Real populations are certainly not homogeneous, but they can be considered as made up of homogeneous groups, each represented by one or more couples. The preliminary study of homogeneous groups is therefore not without interest; besides, it is essential when one cannot formulate analytic approaches to heterogeneity and is obliged to construct a heterogeneous group as a combination of homogeneous groups. This is the situation in which we find ourselves.

In the absence of intra-uterine mortality, the distribution of conceptions by the duration of marriage assumes certain patterns (cf. Appendix 1). In principle, one could therefore conclude, in the presence of deviations from these expectations, that intra-uterine mortality exists, even without direct data on this topic. In practice, such deviations may very easily occur by chance, because they depend on differences and even on second order differences between successive observations.

In addition, if one tries to study empirical data directly, without any hypothesis regarding the distribution of fecundability, it is clear that observed data can be explained without recourse to intra-uterine mortality, by operating solely on the distribution of fecundability.

Consequently, one cannot hope to estimate intra-uterine mortality by observations on only the distributions of first births by the duration of marriage. However, in the knowledge that intra-uterine mortality exists at a fairly high level, it is not without interest to study how such mortality would modify theoretical distributions, according to a hypothesis, which is *a priori* acceptable, regarding to the distribution of fecundabilty.

AVAILABLE DATA

Results from models can be compared with observations either after completing the study of models or as one goes along. After having leaned, in turn, in favor of each one of these two approaches, we prefer the second because it allows us to eliminate certain cases and thus lightens the labor.

A good system of registration of births is required for deriving a distribution of first births by the duration of marriage in months. Since such information is not generally available for pop-

TABLE 3

DISTRIBUTION OF FIRST LIVE BIRTHS
BY DURATION OF MARRIAGE
FOR HISTORICAL AND MODERN GROUPS

Duration of Marriage		Historical Data				Modern Group		
In Completed Months	Less 9 Months	Live Births	q per 1,000	r per 1,000		Live Births	q per 1,000	r per 1,000
				Crude	Adjusted*			
8		105				674		
9	0	281	195			1,444	220	
10	1	217	187	772	770	1,110	217	769
11	2	121	128	558	560	766	192	690
12	3	110	133	909	850	586	181	765
13	4	91	127	827	——	439	166	749
14	5	68	109	747	860	337	153	768
15	6	60	108	882	——	255	136	757
16	7	63	127	1,050	870	213	132	836
17	8	43	99	683	——	186	133	873
18	9	37	95	860	880	144	118	774
19	10	29	82	784	——	117	109	813
20	11	30	93	1,035		115	120	983
21	12	19	65	633		104	124	905
22	13	19	69	1,000		93	126	894
23	14	20	78	1,052		66	103	710
24 plus		236				577		
Total		1,549				7,226		

*Adjusted graphically.

ulations whose fertility has remained natural or almost so, it is hardly astonishing that only a very small number of applicable observations are available. The largest collection of data is that studied by Vincent [1]: it consists of the first postmarital concep- tions of 7,226 women, of whom 6,552 had not yet been confined exactly nine months after the marriage. This collection of data has two disadvantages: (a) it is selected, since all of these women had at least nine live births; (b) more than 20 percent of these women were married before the age of 19; for them, fecundabil- ity increased following marriage. Therefore the conditions do not hold completely, but we may assume that, for a few months, the situation is not too far from that in the models.

There are other sets of observations relating to historic popula- tions: French Canadians (Henripin [1]), bourgeois of Geneva (Henry [3]), villagers of Crulai (Gautier and Henry [1]) and of the three parishes of the "pays de Thelle" (Ganiage [2]), and

TABLE 4

VALUES OF THE TWO INDICES CALCULATED ON THE BASIS
OF V CONCEPTIONS (q_c AND $1 - r_c$)
AND OF BIRTHS (q_b AND $1 - r_b$)
—BASED ON VINCENT'S MODEL

Conceptions			Births		
Duration of Marriage to Conception (Months)	q_c	$1 - r_c$	Marriage Duration (Months)	q_b	$1 - r_b$
0	251		9	220	
1	220	343	10	218	227
2	198	298	11	196	297
3	181	267	12	179	265
4	167	244	13	165	243
5	155	227	14	153	225
6	145	209	15	144	203
7	137	192	16	136	191
8	130	181	17	129	180
9	144	170	18	123	169

Italians of Tunis (Ganiage [1]). Each series contains only a few women and chance fluctuations are obvious. It was therefore necessary to combine them into one rather heterogeneous group that is still considerably less numerous than Vincent's group. It consists of the first post-marital conceptions of 1,549 women of whom 1,444 had still not been confined exactly nine months after marriage; less than a quarter the size of Vincent's sample. This historical group was not selected, but it does include women married before maturity. Thus, it does have one of the two disadvantages of Vincent's data, but fortunately the less important disadvantage.

Table 3 shows, for the two sets of data, the distribution of first live births by the duration of marriage in completed months, as well as the monthly fertility rate, q, and the monthly V conception ratio, r.

When the data are charted (Figures 1 and 2), certain difficulties in the comparison of observations and models are suggested. Chance fluctuations certainly exist in q; in r they are so marked in the case of the historical data that one is not very sure that the adjustment we have attempted has any value. Nevertheless, we will try to extract what we can from these data.

These observations pertain to live births whose timing within marriage is influenced by the timing of marriage in the ovarian cycle, and by the duration of pregnancy. But these considerations

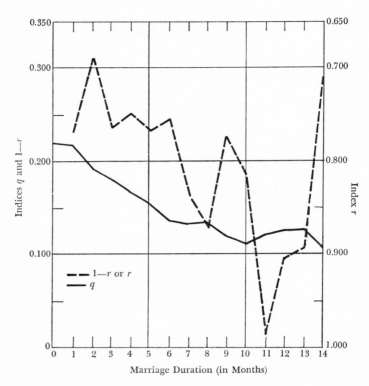

Figure 1. Indices, by month of marriage, as calculated from data for the modern group.

affect only the first values of q and $1 - r$, as is shown by Table 4, which is based on calculations published by Vincent.[7] [For the purposes of this paragraph we denote the indices respectively defined in Eqs. (1) and (2) and relating to conceptions by the subscript c. Corresponding indices relating to births will be denoted by the subscript b.] As seen in Table 4, except for the first month the indices q_b and $1 - r_b$ are approximately equal to the corresponding indices q_c and $1 - r_c$ that relate to V conceptions that occurred nine months earlier. The comparison of models and observations separated by nine months is therefore perfectly justified except for the first month.

---

[7] Vincent ([1], p. 207, Table XXXVI) formulated a model where [two-fifths of −L.H.] the marriages took place before ovulation and [three-fifths −L.H.] some days after ovulation, and calculated q_b according to q_c. We have calculated $1 - r_c$ and $1 - r_b$ from q_c and q_b.

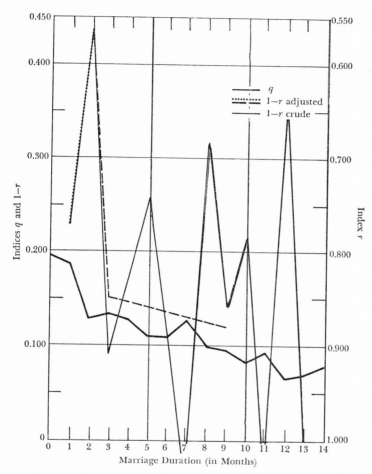

Figure 2. Values of q and $1—r$ by month of marriage as calculated from historical data.

HOMOGENEOUS GROUPS

Using the method described in Appendix 2, we have calculated q assuming an intra-uterine mortality of 25 percent, various values of fecundability and two durations of the nonsusceptible period related to A conceptions: one short, equal to the duration of pregnancy plus one month, and the other long, equal to the duration of pregnancy plus three months. Table 5 and Figures 3 and 4 show the results obtained.

TABLE 5

MONTHLY FERTILITY RATES q (PER 1,000 WOMEN),
BY DURATION OF MARRIAGE
FOR SHORT AND LONG NONSUSCEPTIBLE PERIODS
AND VARIOUS LEVELS OF FECUNDABILITY

Marriage Duration (Months)	Short Nonsusceptible Period							Long Nonsusceptible Period		
	Fecundability							Fecundability		
	0.05	0.15	0.25	0.35	0.45	0.55	0.65	0.15	0.25	0.35
0	375	1,125	1,875	2,625	3,375	4,125	4,875	1,125	1,875	2,625
1	370	1,077	1,730	2,312	2,801	3,160	3,329	1,077	1,730	2,312
2	365	1,026	1,570	1,958	2,140	2,077	1,746	1,026	1,570	1,958
3	362	999	1,491	1,864	1,961	2,001	2,034	972	1,396	1,582
4	360	987	1,461	1,785	1,993	2,167	2,375	915	1,216	1,222
5	360	985	1,463	1,811	2,079	2,326	2,560	891	1,156	1,216
6	361	981	1,460	1,804	2,068	2,261	2,354	883	1,177	1,332
7	361	979	1,456	1,797	2,040	2,195	2,257	886	1,223	1,482
8	358	979	1,452	1,789	2,016	2,151	2,225	889	1,246	1,538
9	359	978	1,447	1,776	2,005	2,149	2,266	891	1,256	1,530
10	359	976	1,446	1,772	2,013	2,211	2,313	891	1,254	1,482
11	360	976	1,454	1,801	2,033	2,275	2,406	888	1,240	1,439
12	360	978	1,453	1,808	2,061	2,244	2,340	888	1,235	1,436
13	359	977	1,453	1,794	2,005	2,218	2,266	892	1,236	1,462
14	358	982	1,449	1,799	2,026	2,222	2,293	892	1,243	1,473

In the absence of intra-uterine mortality, the monthly fertility rate would be constant because of assumed homogeneity. Intra-uterine mortality at first lowers this rate; the decrease is rapid and lasts at least until women whose first conception is an A conception have not yet emerged from the corresponding non-susceptible period.[8] After the phase of decreasing values, the rates present damped oscillations. With a short nonsusceptible period, the oscillations are noticeable only in the case of very high fecund-

---

[8] At the beginning of month n, a proportion $(1 - p)^n$ of the women are expected not to have conceived at all; $1 - (1 - p)^n$ to have conceived only once when n is sufficiently small so that no one has as yet emerged from the nonsusceptible period. Among these conceptions there are $v - v(1 - p)^n$ V conceptions. Hence the proportion of women who have not yet had a V conception is $1 - v + v(1 - p)^n$. During month n the number of expected conceptions is $p(1 - p)^n$, of which $vp(1 - p)^n$ are V conceptions. One then has:

$$q = p \, \frac{v(1 - p)^n}{v(1 - p)^n + 1 - v} = p \, \frac{1}{1 + \dfrac{1 - v}{v(1 - p)^n}};$$

q decreases as n increases.

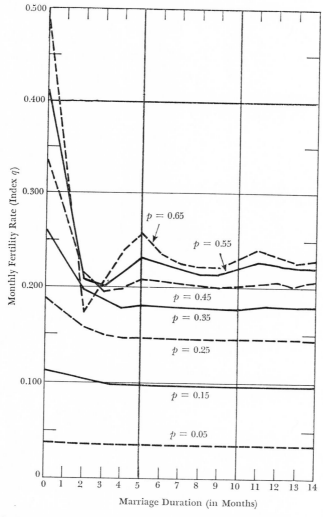

Figure 3. Monthly fertility rate for $v = 0.75$ by different values of fecundability p. Homogeneous groups. Short nonsusceptible period.

ability; with a long nonsusceptible period, they are obvious even for moderate levels of fecundability.

Let us compare these findings to the observations. At first it appears that the historical data show the larger oscillations that are related to long nonsusceptible periods; but this first impres-

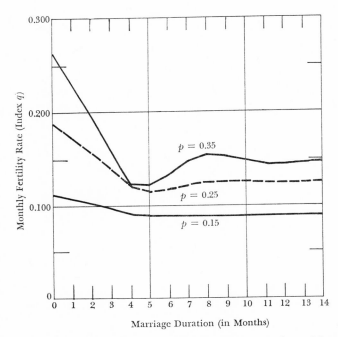

Figure 4. Monthly fertility rate for $v = 0.75$, by different values of fecundability p. Homogeneous groups. Long nonsusceptible periods.

sion is deceptive. The oscillations in Figure 2 start much too early (the reversal occurs at two months as for short monsusceptible periods) to be due to long nonsusceptible periods, and their amplitude is too great for short nonsusceptible periods. Sampling variations are probably responsible for these phenomena. On the other hand, there is nothing against our considering the time of reversal, between two and three months, as an indicator of a predominance of short nonsusceptible periods, the amplitude of the oscillations being, in this case, an effect of chance.

In the two observed groups, the value of the fertility rate, q, does not level off as it does in the models. The rapid decrease in the first months is followed by a less rapid decrease, which still remains considerable.

Hence, real groups cannot be homogeneous at the same time for all three fundamental characteristics: fecundability, duration of nonsusceptibility and intra-uterine mortality. It is only in the very early months that the existence of intra-uterine mortality

TABLE 6

MONTHLY FERTILITY RATES, q (PER 1,000),
FOR A GROUP WITH HETEROGENEOUS NONSUSCEPTIBLE PERIODS,
BY DURATION OF MARRIAGE AND FECUNDABILITY

Month	$p = 0.25$	$p = 0.35$	Month	$p = 0.25$	$p = 0.35$
0	187.5	262.5	8	134	165
1	173	231	9	134	163.5
2	157	196	10	134	160
3	144.5	170	11	134	159
4	134	150	12	133	159
5	131	150	13	133	159
6	131	155	14	133	160
7	133	162			

produces, in homogeneous groups, a decrease in the monthly fertility rate. Until now, one has tended to interpret this early decrease as a consequence of heterogeneous fecundability; in fact, it is the continuation of the decrease after these first months that is the sign of heterogeneity in observed groups.

Let use now examine the effects of heterogeneity in each one of the fundamental characteristics.

HETEROGENEITY OF THE DURATION
OF NONSUSCEPTIBILITY

Let us form a heterogeneous group by combining, in equal proportions, groups with long and short nonsusceptible periods, with fecundabilities close to the average, 0.25 and 0.35. One obtains the results shown in Table 6 and Figure 5. The heterogeneous groups are not different from the homogeneous groups of which they are composed: the fertility rate seems to become stabilized following damped oscillations.

In principle, however, the rate q ought to be decreasing continually. It is a weighted mean of two rates, each of which tends to become stabilized. The weights change over time, the rate for the subgroup with a long nonsusceptible period being weighted relatively more as the duration of observations increases. Therefore, the mean rate should be continually approaching the lower rate, i.e. that of the subgroup with the longer duration of nonsusceptibility. But since the difference between the extreme values

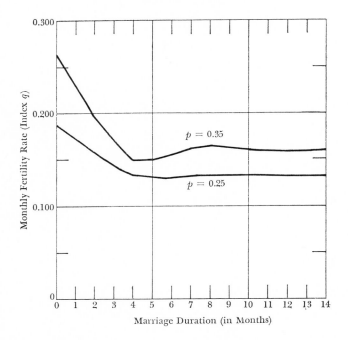

Figure 5. Monthly fertility rate for $v = 0.75$, by different values of fecundability p. Group heterogeneous for duration of nonsusceptibility.

of the rate is small, the decrease is slow and passes unnoticed, especially in view of the oscillations.

The heterogeneous groups that we have constructed are probably more heterogeneous than any real population; the oscillations are in fact shifted more to the right than in the two observed groups. Heterogeneity limited to the nonsusceptible period after intra-uterine death therefore cannot alone explain the continuing decrease in the fertility rate q that is observed in real populations.

In real populations, heterogeneity must also exist either in fecundability alone, in intra-uterine mortality alone or in both. One can, however, eliminate the case with homogeneous fecundability and heterogeneous intra-uterine mortality because a comparison of fertility rates q and the corresponding quantities $1 - r$, shows that real groups are heterogeneous in fecundability (Appendix 4).

HETEROGENEITY IN FECUNDABILITY

I. WITHOUT INTRA-UTERINE MORTALITY

We have assumed that the distribution of fecundability is approximately of a Pearson type I. With such a distribution, the monthly fertility rate at month n is of the form:

$$q = \frac{a}{a + b + n}$$

where a and b are the parameters of the distribution (see Appendix 3, Eq. (A22)). As shown in Eq. (A24) and (A25),

$$1 - r = \frac{a + 1}{a + b + n},$$

and the ratio:

$$\frac{1 - r}{q} = 1 + \frac{1}{a},$$

is constant.

Let us see what becomes of these relations for the simplified distributions that we use in the numerical calculations (for definitions, see Appendix 4).

Distribution A. This distribution (see Table A3) includes seven values of fecundability, with a mean of 0.32 and the squared coefficient of variation (c^2) equal to 0.313. The ratio $(1 - r)/q$ varies little and is equal on the average to 1.57 during months 1-14. This value of the ratio corresponds to a value of the parameter a very close to 1.75; if one associates it with a value of the parameter b equal to 3.75, one obtains a Pearson type I distribution with a mean of 0.318 and a value of c^2 equal to 0.330. The values of q and of $1 - r$ that correspond to this type I distribution are very close to those of distribution A, as can be seen in Table 7 and Figure 6.

Distribution B. In distribution B (see Appendix 4) consisting of six fecundabilities with identical frequencies, we have deliberately departed considerably from Pearson type I distributions. The ratio $[(1 - r)/q$ —L.H.] varies a great deal more than was the case for distribution A. In months two to fourteen, however, as seen in Table 8, it does not deviate more than 7 percent from the mean for the first fourteen months, 1.73. Again one obtains a

TABLE 7
VALUES OF q, $1 - r$, AND $(1 - r)/q$ (PER 1,000)
BY DURATION OF MARRIAGE FOR TWO DISTRIBUTIONS
OF FECUNDABILITY (DISTRIBUTION A AND PEARSON I)

Month	Distribution A			Pearson I: $a = 1.75$ $b = 3.75$		
	q	$1 - r$	$(1-r)/q$	q	$1 - r$	$(1-r)/q$
0	320			318		
1	273	420	1.54	269	423	1.57
2	236	371	1.57	233	369	id.
3	207	328	1.58	206	324	id.
4	185	293	1.58	184	290	id.
5	167	264	1.58	167	262	id.
6	152	240	1.58	152	239	id.
7	140	221	1.58	140	220	id.
8	130	204	1.57	130	204	id.
9	121	190	1.57	121	190	id.
10	113	178	1.58	113	178	id.
11	106	166	1.57	106	167	id.
12	100	157	1.57	100	157	id.
13	95	148	1.56	95	149	id.
14	90	140	1.56	90	141	id.

good approximation to the series of the rates q and the quantities $1 - r$ using a Pearson type I distribution having the parameters $a = 1.36$, $b = 3.04$ (mean fecundability $= 0.309$, $c^2 = 0.414$), as is shown in Table 8 and Figure 7.

Thus, in the absence of intra-uterine mortality, the fertility rates q and the quantities $1 - r$ would have similar properties to those produced in the case where fecundability is distributed as in a Pearson type I: curves of q and of $1 - r$, which are strictly parallel on a semi-log graph and appear parallel also on an ordinary graph, which show progressive diminution in the slope, and a ratio $(1 - r)/q$ that varies little, if at all, in practice.

Reference to Figures 1 and 2 will confirm, especially for the historical data, that the real observations are quite different from these characteristics of heterogeneous groups without intra-uterine mortality. Instead of decreasing progressively, the slope is abruptly interrupted; instead of remaining parallel to the fertility rate, the curve of $1 - r$ seems to plunge towards it.

II. UNIFORM INTRA-UTERINE MORTALITY

Assuming the same distributions of fecundability, A and B, we will add uniform intra-uterine mortalities ranging from 15

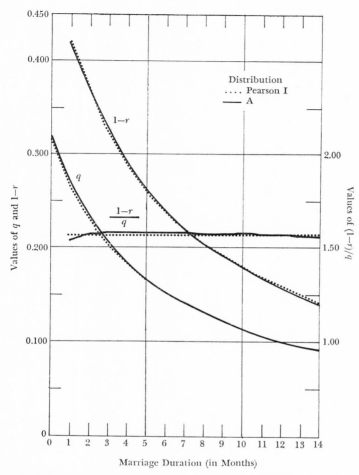

Figure 6. Values of q, $1-r$, and $(1-r)/q$ for two distributions (Pearson type I and A) of fecundability. Heterogeneous groups. Intra-uterine mortality 0.

percent to 50 percent. The resulting values of q, $1 - r$ and $[(1 - r)/q -L.H.]$ are shown in Tables 9 and 10.

Figure 8 to 13 which are based on these tables bring out a number of interesting results.

1. For a given value of intra-uterine mortality, the three curves representing q, $1 - r$, and $(1 - r)/q$ for distribution A differ little from the corresponding curves for distribution B. Since (except for the mean and the variance) distributions A and B differ appreciably from each other, it seems reasonable to con-

TABLE 8

VALUES OF q, $1 - r$, AND $(1 - r)/q$ (PER 1,000)
BY DURATION OF MARRIAGE FOR TWO DISTRIBUTIONS
OF FECUNDABILITY (DISTRIBUTION B AND PEARSON I)

Month	Distribution B			Pearson I: $a = 1.36$ $b = 3.04$		
	q	$1-r$	$(1-r)/q$	q	$1-r$	$(1-r)/q$
0	300			309		
1	258	397	1.54	252	437	1.735
2	221	365	1.65	212.5	369	id.
3	190	331	1.74	184	319	id.
4	165	297	1.80	162	281	id.
5	145	266	1.83	145	251	id.
6	129	238	1.84	131	227	id.
7	117	215	1.84	119	207	id.
8	107	193	1.80	110	190	id.
9	98.5	176	1.79	101	176	id.
10	92	159	1.73	94.5	164	id.
11	86	147	1.70	88	153	id.
12	81.5	137	1.68	83	144	id.
13	77.5	126	1.63	78	136	id.
14	74	119	1.61	74	128	id.

clude that when we know the mean and the variance of fecundability, the other characteristics of the distribution are of little importance, except, perhaps, if a distribution deviates even further from distribution A than does distribution B.

2. Again one sees, even for relatively low levels of intra-uterine mortality, the inflections in the curves of the fertility rates q, and of $1 - r$ already noticed in homogeneous groups. But here, the early rapid decrease is followed by a long phase of decelerated decrease, and not by a long plateau. With very high intra-uterine mortality, however, the decline in q is slight and that in $1 - r$ is not marked, so that, in this case, the contrast with homogeneous groups seems to disappear. The contrast does, however, exist in the ratio $(1 - r)/q$, since this ratio remains greater than 1, while in homogeneous groups it oscillates around one.[9]

---

[9] The diminution in the slope at the right hand side of the curves of q, as intra-uterine mortality increases, seen in Figure 8 and 9, may be explained as follows. The fertility rate of a heterogeneous group is a weighted mean of the rates of the subgroups of which it is composed, the weights being the subjects that remain (those who have not yet had a V conception). In the absence of intra-uterine mortality, there is a rapid selection of the less fecundable women and the rate decreases continuously. With high intra-uterine mortality, on the contrary, the relative difference between the numbers remaining decreases much less quickly. For example, given an original group

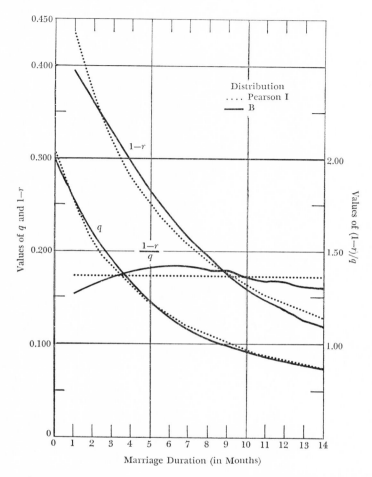

Figure 7. Values of q, $1-r$, and $(1-r)/q$ for two distributions (Pearson type I and B) of fecundability. Heterogeneous groups. Intra-uterine mortality 0.

---

of 10,000 women, half of whom have a fecundability of 0.25 and half have a fecundability of 0.35, the numbers without a V conception at the end of 14 months is:

Fecundability	Intra-Uterine Mortality	
	0 percent	50 percent
0.25	133	2471
0.35	14	1755

Without intra-uterine mortality, the mean fecundability at fifteen months is close to 0.26; with a mortality of 50 percent it is still a little above 0.29, in comparison with a rate of 0.30 in both cases at month zero.

TABLE 9

VALUES OF q, $1-r$, AND $(1-r)/q$ (PER 1,000) BY DURATION OF MARRIAGE FOR VARIOUS LEVELS OF INTRA-UTERINE MORTALITY AND FECUNDABILITY. DISTRIBUTION A

Month	Intra-Uterine Motality 15 Percent			Intra-Uterine Mortality 25 Percent			Intra-Uterine Mortality 35 Percent			Intra-Uterine Mortality 50 Percent		
	q	$1-r$	$(1-r)/q$	q	$1-r$	$(1-r)/q$	q	$1-r$	$(1-r)/q$	q	$1-r$	$(1-r)/q$
0	272			240			208			160		
1	217	420	1.94	183	420	2.30	152	420	2.76	110	420	3.82
2	174	371	2.13	141	371	2.63	113	371	3.28	78	371	4.76
3	158	248	1.57	132	197	1.49	109	143	1.31	79	62	0.78
4	150	200	1.33	130	147	1.13	110	101	0.92	82	44	0.54
5	145	180	1.24	128	142	1.11	110	111	1.01	83	76	0.92
6	137	194	1.42	122	169	1.39	105	148	1.41	79	122	1.54
7	130	180	1.38	117	159	1.36	101	136	1.35	77	104	1.35
8	122	179	1.47	112	153	1.37	99	128	1.29	76	89	1.17
9	117	162	1.38	108	144	1.33	96	123	1.28	75	90	1.20
10	111	158	1.42	104	138	1.33	93	120	1.29	74	92	1.24
11	106	155	1.46	101	129	1.28	92	105	1.14	73	80	1.10
12	102	139	1.36	97	137	1.41	89	122	1.37	72	91	1.26
13	96	155	1.61	93	136	1.46	86	119	1.38	70	96	1.37
14	92	130	1.41	89	130	1.46	84	107	1.39	69	79	1.14

TABLE 10

VALUES OF q, $1 - r$, AND $(1 - r)/q$ (PER 1,000) BY DURATION OF MARRIAGE
FOR VARIOUS LEVELS OF INTRA-UTERINE MORTALITY AND FECUNDABILITY. DISTRIBUTION B

Month	Intra-Uterine Mortality 15 Percent			Intra-Uterine Mortality 25 Percent			Intra-Uterine Mortality 35 Percent			Intra-Uterine Mortality 50 Percent		
	q	$1-r$	$(1-r)/q$	q	$1-r$	$(1-r)/q$	q	$1-r$	$(1-r)/q$	q	$1-r$	$(1-r)/q$
0	255			225			195			150		
1	206	397	1.93	175	397	2.27	146	397	2.72	106	397	3.74
2	165	364	2.21	135	364	2.70	109	364	3.34	76	364	4.79
3	147	259	1.76	123	211	1.72	102	163	1.60	74	92	1.24
4	137	203	1.48	119	150	1.26	102	104	1.02	77	44	0.57
5	130	179	1.38	116	138	1.19	102	104	1.02	78	66	0.85
6	122	188	1.54	110	162	1.47	97	145	1.49	74	116	1.57
7	114	176	1.54	105	153	1.46	91	131	1.44	72	102	1.42
8	106	173	1.63	99	152	1.53	89	128	1.44	71	92	1.30
9	101	156	1.54	95	137	1.44	87	117	1.35	69	92	1.33
10	95	149	1.57	91	139	1.53	84	118	1.40	68	82	1.21
11	90	144	1.60	88	121	1.47	81	107	1.32	67	86	1.28
12	86	130	1.51	84	123	1.46	78	115	1.47	66	82	1.24
13	80	150	1.87	80	134	1.67	75	115	1.53	63	88	1.40
14	76	126	1.66	76	122	1.60	73	107	1.47	62	85	1.37

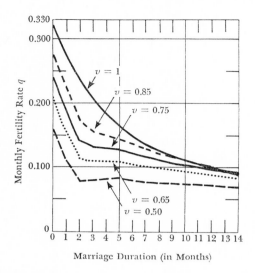

Figure 8. Monthly fertility rates according to intra-uterine mortality. Heterogeneous group. Distribution A.

Available observations depart appreciably from this case, since the curve of the fertility rates continues to go down. One concludes from this that the observed groups could not have had intra-uterine mortality rates which were at the same time both very high and uniform. But, if the mean intra-uterine mortality is very high, its dispersion cannot be great, so that one must take it as likely that considerably fewer than half the conceptions are A conceptions followed by a nonsusceptible period. In other words, if intra-uterine mortality in the first month of pregnancy (in the usual sense) is as high as certain observations suggest, it must very frequently occur so early that no nonsusceptible period results, i.e. there is neither a noticeable delay in menses nor a higher frequency of anovulation in the next cycle. As far as the delay in menses is concerned, this conclusion is supported by another argument. Pregnancies resulting in very early intra-uterine mortality often pass unnoticed; this would not be the case if there were an interruption of menses, even for only one month.

3. The curve of the fertility rates for intra-uterine mortality levels of 15–25 percent closely resembles that observed in the historical data. (Figures 8 and 9 as compared with Figure 2.) Some

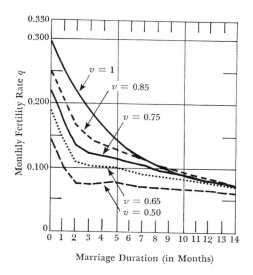

Figure 9. Monthly fertility rates according to intra-uterine mortality. Heterogeneous group. Distribution B.

similarity may also exist in the curves of the quantities $1 - r$. (Figures 10 and 11.) In the historical data (Figure 2), as in the models, $1 - r$ is at first much higher than q, then drops, approaching q, stops a little above it and then descends in an almost completely parallel curve.[10]

The modern group (Figure 1) does not resemble the models developed up to this point. The curve of the fertility rates would be better fitted by three linear segments than by two (from 0–2 months, from 2–6 and after 6); the curve of $1 - r$, from month two to month three, approaches that of the fertility rate, but much less closely than in the models; it then remains horizontal or almost so, for several months. To be sure, it is not impossible that chance fluctuations affect the observations in a large group more than in a small group; the reverse is, however, more likely. We ought, consequently, to try to explain why the modern group departs from a model which would appear to provide a good fit to the historical data.

---

[10] In theory, the similarity of the rates ought to imply a similarity of the quantities $1 - r$; but the chance fluctuations in the latter, which are greater, may easily mask the resemblances.

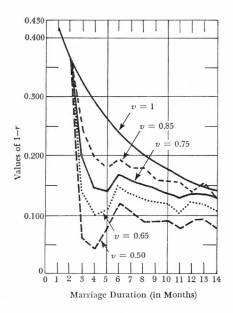

Figure 10. Values of $1-r$ according to intra-uterine mortality. Heterogeneous group. Distribution A.

III. HETEROGENEITY OF INTRA-UTERINE MORTALITY

The fact that spontaneous abortions are less frequent when the previous pregnancy ended in a live birth than in the opposite case is undoubtedly due, in large part, to the inequality of the risks of spontaneous abortion between women.[11] It is necessary, therefore, to study the effect of this inequality of the risks on variations in q, $1-r$ and the ratio $(1-r)/q$, with the duration of marriage.

To go on to this study it is necessary to have some idea of the dispersion of the risk of spontaneous abortion. One can evaluate it, at least approximately, from available data on the frequency of spontaneous abortions according to the outcome of the preceding pregnancy, by live birth or spontaneous abortion. This is what we have done in Appendix 5, according to data obtained in the United States. Having estimated the dispersion, we have calculated an appropriate distribution of the probability v that

---

[11] The risk can also vary for the same woman and can increase, particularly during a specified period after each spontaneous abortion. On this subject, see D. Warburton and F. C. Fraser [1].

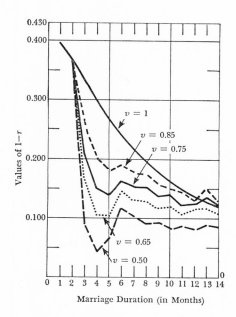

Figure 11. Values of 1—r according to intra-uterine mortality. Heterogeneous group. Distribution B.

a conception ends in a live birth, assuming that this distribution was of a Pearson type I. As in the case of fecundability, we have replaced it by a simplified distribution that includes only seven values, between 0.65 and 0.95 (see Appendix 5, Table A4).

Assuming that fecundability and intra-uterine mortality are independent, we have calculated monthly fertility rates in a model heterogeneous in two respects, fecundability with distribution A, and the probability v with the distribution defined above.

One thus obtains the results shown in Table 11. Figure 14, which is based on this table, shows that the characteristics of the curves obtained with uniform intra-uterine mortality persist when the variation in intra-uterine mortality is of the order of magnitude of the variation that exists in reality.[12]

We confirm, as before, that the historical data conforms to

---

[12] We first made trials with a distribution of $(1 - v)$ limited to two values: 0 and twice the mean value. In this case, the results are substantially different from the above; in particular, the curve of the rates cannot be assimilated to a broken line formed from two straight lines.

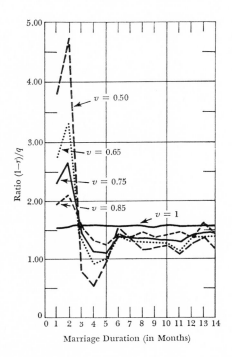

Figure 12. Values of the ratio $(1-r)/q$ according to intra-uterine mortality. Heterogeneous group. Distribution A.

this model. This result is satisfying; since it is unlikely that a human group would be homogeneous with respect to any quality, it would have been deceptive to obtain a good approximation to reality with a homogeneous model and to lose it on passing to a heterogeneous model.

SPECIAL INVESTIGATION
OF THE MODERN GROUP

This satisfaction is, however, moderated by the failure of the models with respect to the modern group, which is the most numerous. Since this group differs from the historical data by the fact that it includes only women who had many births, let us see what effects this selection could have on this group. First, among women who have just conceived their first child, the

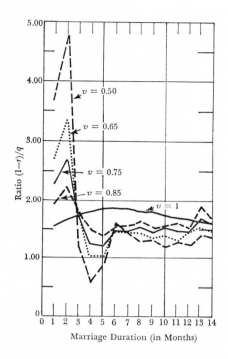

Figure 13. Values of the ratio $(1-r)/q$ according to intra-uterine mortality. Heterogeneous group. Distribution B.

proportion who will have at least eight other births decreases as the duration of marriage increases, and, according to models studied a few years ago,[13] the monthly fertility rate of a group with uniform fecundability increases rather than remaining constant. This increase, however, remains small during a relatively short period of time.

The proportion of women who will have nine births increases with increasing fecundability. The selected group is, therefore, different from the initial group. If mean fecundability is higher, fecundability is less dispersed.

These results of selection have the effect only of reducing the

---

[13] [See Chapter Three, Table 6. These data allow the calculation of fertility rates by quarter for families with nine children; the procedure is as follows: cumulate the figures in column $C_{9,1}$ from the end and then divide each of the figures in column $C_{9,1}$ by the corresponding cumulative total, for example, 1713 by 3459, 874 by 1746, ...]

TABLE 11

VALUES OF q, $1 - r$, AND $(1 - r)/q$ (PER 1,000)
BY DURATION OF MARRIAGE IN A HETEROGENEOUS MODEL
WITH FECUNDABILITY DISTRIBUTION A
AND A HETEROGENEOUS DISTRIBUTION
FOR INTRA-UTERINE MORTALITY

Month	q	$1 - r$	$(1 - r)/q$	Month	q	$1 - r$	$(1 - r)/q$
0	261			8	116	167	1.44
1	205	420	2.05	9	111	155	1.40
2	162	371	2.29	10	106	148	1.40
3	148	235	1.59	11	102	138	1.35
4	141	186	1.32	12	98	138	1.41
5	136	169	1.24	13	94	142	1.51
6	129	185	1.43	14	90	128	1.42
7	122	172	1.41				

slope of the right hand side of the curve of monthly fertility rates. They could not therefore explain the difference between the modern group and the models.

Women who are most exposed to the risk of spontaneous abortion have the least chance of having nine births or more; the selected group therefore has a higher mean value of the probability v and a smaller dispersion than those with fewer births. In addition, a woman has more chances of having many births if she has, at the same time, both high fecundability and a low risk of intra-uterine mortality. Selection certainly has the effect of eliminating women of low fecundability who have, at the same time, high risks of spontaneous abortion. Hence, curves such as those in Figure 3 would be less dispersed than if there were no selection. This constriction also contributes to reducing the slope of the curve of fertility rates. Again, this effect is not what we are seeking.

Selection has, however, another effect that we must now examine: it decreases the mean risk of spontaneous abortion. Now, the break in the slope of the curve of the fertility rates, q, exists only when intra-uterine mortality is sufficiently high. For a sufficiently low intra-uterine mortality, the curve of monthly fertility rates may then resemble that of the modern group. In addition, Vincent ([1], p. 207) developed a model which resembles that of

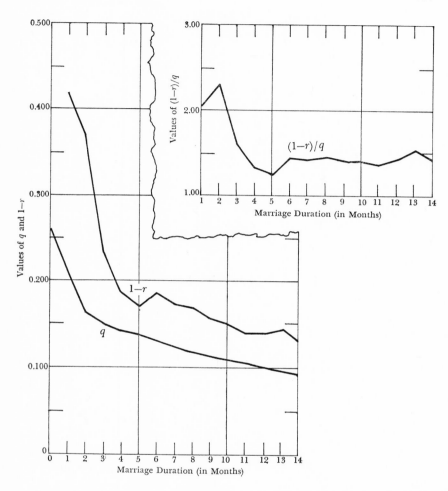

Figure 14. Value of q, $1-r$, and $(1-r)/q$. Group heterogeneous for fecundability and intra-uterine mortality.

a group having zero intra-uterine mortality and which is heterogeneous with respect to fecundability.[14]

At first glance, however, it is not clear how selection could almost completely eliminate women predisposed to spontaneous

[14] The inverse of the quotient is, for several months, almost a linear function of the duration of marriage. Now, one finds a linear relation between the inverse of the rate and the duration, if fecundability is distributed according to the Pearson type I curve (see Appendix 3, Eq. (A22)).

TABLE 12

MONTHLY FERTILITY RATES, q (PER 1,000),

BY DURATION OF MARRIAGE

FOR TWO LEVELS OF INTRA-UTERINE MORTALITY $(1 - v)$

FOR THE FIRST PREGNANCY AND A CLUSTER EFFECT

Month	Intra-Uterine Mortality for the First Pregnancy		Month	Intra-Uterine Mortality for the First Pregnancy	
	0.15	0.25		0.15	0.25
0	272	240	8	113	89
1	217	183	9	109	86
2	174	141	10	105	83
3	155	124	11	99	81
4	144	115	12	96	78
5	136	108	13	92	74
6	127	100	14	89	72
7	120	94			

abortions while permitting the retention of women of low fecundability. If intra-uterine mortality were not accompanied by a nonsusceptible period, the selection would not have a greater effect on women with fecundability equal to .40 and a probability v equal to .50 than on those having a fecundability of 0.20 and a probability v of 1. The existence of a nonsusceptible period after conception makes such a difference possible; but, since the nonsusceptible period is short, one doubts that this would greatly reduce the mean frequency of spontaneous abortions in a selected group.

It could perhaps be otherwise, if intra-uterine mortality were considerably increased for several months following a spontaneous abortion (cluster effect). Women characterized by high intra-uterine mortality would then have only a small chance of having many children (similar to women with a long nonsusceptible period). One can, however, accept this hypothesis only if it does not modify too greatly the curve of [fertility] rates, in the absence of selection, since the models where intra-uterine mortality is identical before and after an intra-uterine death do provide a good fit to the observations on the historical data.

To examine this point, we have calculated monthly fertility rates, for the case where intra-uterine mortality would be doubled

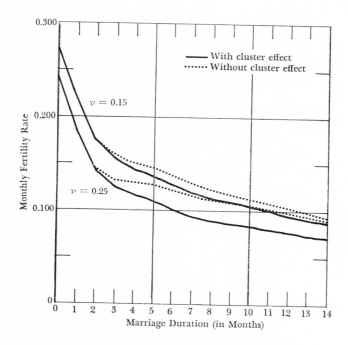

Figure 15. Monthly fertility rate with and without cluster effect, for two levels of intra-uterine mortality.

during at least 13 months following a spontaneous abortion.[15] The values of the monthly rates (for intra-uterine mortality of 0.15 to 0.25 during the first pregnancy) are shown in Table 12.

A graphic comparison (Figure 15) of these series and those obtained in the case where intra-uterine mortality is not affected by the outcome of the preceding pregnancy, shows that the cluster effect blurs the break in the slope observed previously and produces more continuous variations in the curve. This change is, on reflection, a logical result of the assumed increase in intra-uterine mortality in the months that follow a spontaneous abortion. As a result of this increase, the probability of V_1 conceptions[16] is less than it would be without the cluster effect, while

---

[15] For reasons of convenience, we have chosen 13 months rather than 12; with 13 the higher mortality occurs until the end of the 15 month period studied. The method of calculation is that of Appendix 2, "Change in Mortality after the First Intra-Uterine Death."

[16] We denote by V_k a V conception preceded by k A conceptions.

the probability of V_2 conceptions is greater. This tends to lower the curve in its middle part and raise it more at the right.

Curves deformed in this way by the cluster effect still show a good fit to the historical data. In those data, chance fluctuations are, in fact, noticeably too great to allow us to decide whether the shape of the curve of fertility rates is that of the model with the cluster effect or that of the model without the cluster effect.

It then would not be impossible that the difference between the historical data and the modern group results from selection, which eliminates (thanks to a marked cluster effect) an important fraction of women characterized by high risks of intra-uterine mortality. Still, there would be necessary, on the one hand, a marked cluster effect, of which we are not confident,[17] and, on the other hand, a knowledge that this effect could produce the strong selection envisioned. This point would alone require a study of models, which, because of its length and complexity, is beyond the range of this article. It is therefore prudent to conclude that perhaps selection explains the very marked difference between the results obtained in the models and the data for the modern group, but that this explanation, at the moment, has only rather weak justification.

SUMMARY

The decrease, with increasing duration of marriage, of monthly fertility rates of women who have not yet borne any children was originally interpreted as a sign of heterogeneity in the fecundability of human groups. Every month mean fecundability is lower than the preceding month, because the proportion of women with high fecundability who have conceived is larger than is the case for those with low fecundability.

The existence of a considerable risk of intra-uterine mortality makes this conclusion less certain. Because of this risk, monthly fertility rates would decrease at the beginning of marriage even in a homogeneous group. The decrease would not continue after the early months unless there is heterogeneity for one of the two fundamental characteristics, fecundability or intra-uterine mortality. Now, in certain available data, the decrease does continue;

---

[17] In the article of Warburton and Fraser [1] already cited, this effect is not statistically significant and the authors consider it weak.

real groups, then, are quite heterogeneous, as previously thought, but not necessarily with respect to fecundability.

In fact, heterogeneity in fecundability does exist and reveals itself in the comparison between fertility rates and $1 - r_{n+1}$, the complement of the ratio r_{n+1} of the V conceptions in month $n + 1$ to those of month n provided that one knows, at least approximately, the mean intra-uterine mortality. In addition, this comparison gives, but with poor precision, an estimate of the dispersion of fecundability.

Heterogeneity of intra-uterine mortality, probable *a priori,* also exists and shows itself by differences in the frequency of spontaneous abortion, depending on whether the preceding pregnancy terminated in a live birth or not. From this difference, one can evaluate the dispersion in intra-uterine mortality.

The comparison between models and observations has given interesting results. They cannot, however, be considered more than presumptions, since the observations in question are not very numerous and since the modern series, the most numerous, is the result of a selection of which one can scarcely know the effect. Here are the presumptions:

(a) The nonsusceptible period that accompanies an A conception (a conception that ends in an intra-uterine death) scarcely lasts longer than one month after the termination of pregnancy, supporting Potter's notions.

(b) If, as is believed, the incidence of intra-uterine deaths before and during implantation is very high, this intra-uterine mortality of the first month differs from that which occurs later by the absence of a nonsusceptible period. Because of this, very early intra-uterine mortality does not play a distinct role, since it can be assimilated to fecundability by giving the latter a more restrictive definition, ignoring A conceptions that are not followed by a nonsusceptible period.

(c) Results obtained with intra-uterine mortality that varies between women do not differ greatly from those given by uniform intra-uterine mortality. In other words, dispersion in intra-uterine mortality does not play an important role in fertility rates at the beginning of marriage. The investigation of models has been facilitated by this finding.

(d) The historical data are very similar to results obtained in models with very high intra-uterine mortality (20 percent to 25 percent), independent of fecundability and without a cluster effect. But, since chance fluctuations remain important, models with a cluster effect also will do; the interest in the latter is not very great since apparently the cluster effect is not great.

(e) The modern group resembles only models with very low intra-uterine mortality. But it is difficult to explain why. More data are therefore indispensable. [A rereading of Chapter 1 of Vincent [1], pp. 24 and 25, shows that he excluded from the analysis a large fraction of women who had spontaneous abortions because of insufficient data. In view of this, it is less surprising that his data resemble only models with very low intra-uterine mortality. —L.H.]

Appendix 1

Let us put the number of couples without prenuptial conceptions equal to unity, and designate by n_0, n_1, ..., n_k, ... expected conceptions occurring in the course of marriage months (equated with cycles) 0, 1, ..., k, ... If $h(p)$ is the probability density of fecundability p, supposedly invariable for each couple, one has:

$$n_0 = \int_0^1 p h(p)\, dp$$

$$n_1 = \int_0^1 p\,(1-p)\, h(p)\, dp$$

$$n_2 = \int_0^1 p\,(1-p)^2\, h(p)\, dp$$

$$n_k = \int_0^1 p\,(1-p)^k\, h(p)\, dp \tag{A1}$$

and thus:

$$n_0 - n_1 = \int_0^1 p^2\, h(p)\, dp$$

$$n_1 - n_2 = \int_0^1 p^2\,(1-p)\, h(p)\, dp$$

$$n_k - n_{k+1} = \int_0^1 p^2\,(1-p)^k\, h(p)\, dp. \tag{A2}$$

The integrals are positive; the successive differences, $n_0 - n_1$, ... are also positive.

In considering the second order differences, one gets:

$$(n_{k-1} - n_k) - (n_k - n_{k+1}) = \int_0^1 p^3 (1-p)^{k-1} h(p)\, dp.$$

$$(A3)$$

The second order differences also are positive, since the integrals are positive. It may be shown progressively that differences of all orders form a decreasing series.

Thus, if a series of conceptions or at least one series of differences of some order is not decreasing, one cannot consider it, except for the effects of chance, as being produced by a group where fecundability is invariant for each couple and where there is no intra-uterine mortality. Since marked variations in fecundability are not to be expected in the course of a few months, one is led to attribute a lack of decrease encountered in a series of differences of some order, if not to chance, then to intra-uterine mortality.

Appendix 2

CALCULATIONS OF V CONCEPTIONS

Monthly V conceptions are the sum of:

V_0, the number of V conceptions that are not preceded by any A conceptions,

V_1, the number of V conceptions that are preceded by one A conception,

V_2, the number of V conceptions that are preceded by two A conceptions, and so on.

We will calculate successively each series. The results for V_0 are obtained most easily: it suffices to multiply v by the number of first conceptions (A and V combined) of the corresponding months. To calculate V_1, we will consider, to begin with, a homogeneous group with fecundability p.

Let us designate by n_i the V conceptions of month i; corresponding to them are $\dfrac{(1-v)\, n_i}{v}$ conceptions of type A. Using the distribution in Table 1, we can estimate that out of these $\dfrac{(1-v)\,n_i}{v}$ conceptions, there are $\dfrac{0.46\,(1-v)\,n_i}{v}$ intra-uterine deaths in month $(i+1)$, $\dfrac{0.26\,(1-v)\,n_i}{v}$ in month $(i+2)$, and so on. Consequently, d_j, the total number of intra-uterine deaths occurring in month j is equal to

$$d_j = \frac{1-v}{v}\,[0.46n_{j-1} + 0.26n_{j-2} + 0.17n_{j-3} + \dots\,].$$
(A4)

Let us denote by a_0, a_1, a_2, ... the number of V conceptions that occur respectively in the course of the months t, $t+1$, $t+2$, ... for women who are susceptible at the beginning of month t.[18]

Assuming that a woman becomes susceptible in the second month after an intra-uterine death, the value of V_1 in month x is then equal to:

$$V_1(x) = a_0 d_{x-2} + a_1 d_{x-3} + a_2 d_{x-4} + \dots + a_k d_{x-k\,2}$$
(A5)

which yields, on substituting the d_j from Eq. (A4):

$$V_1(x) = \frac{(1-v)}{v}\,[a_0(0.46n_{x-3} + 0.26n_{x-4} + 0.17n_{x-5} + \dots)$$
$$+ a_1(0.46n_{x-4} + 0.26n_{x-5} + 0.17n_{x-6} + \dots) + \dots].$$
(A6)

After collecting terms, Eq. (A6) is equal to:

$$V_1(x) = \frac{(1-v)}{v}\Big[\, n_{x-3}\,(0.46a_0) + n_{x-4}(0.46a_1 + 0.26a_0) + \dots$$
$$\dots + n_{x-k}(0.46a_{k-3} + 0.26a_{k-2} + 0.17a_{k-1} + \dots)\,\Big].$$
(A7)

To calculate $V_1(x)$, therefore, we have to determine coefficients α_i:

$$\alpha_0 = \frac{(1-v)}{v} \times 0.46a_0$$

$$\alpha_1 = \frac{(1-v)}{v}\,(0.46a_1 + 0.26a_0)$$

$$\alpha_2 = \frac{(1-v)}{v}\,(0.46a_2 + 0.26a_1 + 0.17a_0).$$
(A8)

---

[18] $a_0 = vp$, $a_1 = vp(1-p)$, $a_2 = vp(1-p)^2 \dots$, $a_k = vp(1-p)^k$.

TABLE A1
VALUES OF c, γ, AND α (PER 10,000)
BY DURATION OF MARRIAGE (IN MONTHS)
FOR A HOMOGENEOUS GROUP

Month of Marriage	c	γ	α	Month of Marriage	c	γ	α
0	3,500	1,610	403	8	112	258	65
1	2,275	1,957	489	9	73	168	42
2	1,479	1,867	467	10	47	109	26
3	961	1,353	338	11	31	71	18
4	625	985	246	12	20	46	11
5	406	675	169	13	13	30	8
6	264	474	118	14	8	19	5
7	172	343	86				

Since these coefficients are independent of the numbers n, they can be used to calculate V_2 from V_1, V_3 from V_2 and so on.

Furthermore, the numbers a_0, a_1, a_2, ... are equal to v times the number of conceptions (A and V combined) c_0, c_1, c_2, ... which are independent of v. Thus, one must first calculate the coefficients γ_i equal to:

$$\gamma_0 = 0.46\, c_0$$

$$\gamma_1 = 0.46\, c_1 + 0.26\, c_0$$

$$\gamma_2 = 0.46\, c_2 + 0.26\, c_1 + 0.17\, c_0$$

$$\text{(A9)}$$

valid for all values of v while the coefficients α correspond to each particular value of v. One has then:

$$\alpha_i = \frac{1-v}{v} \cdot v\gamma_i = (1-v)\,\gamma_i. \qquad \text{(A10)}$$

EXAMPLE

Assume we are concerned with a homogeneous group of 10,000 women with fecundability equal to 0.35, and an intra-uterine mortality of 25 percent. The calculated values of c, γ and α for months 1 to 14 are shown in Table A1.

The results for V_0 to V_3 are shown in Table A2. The calculations can be illustrated as follows: since $n_j = vc_j$, one obtains from Eq. (A7) and the numerical values in Table A1, for example:

TABLE A2

VALUES OF V_0, V_1, V_2, AND V_3

AND THE TOTAL V CONCEPTIONS (BY MONTHS)

Month of Marriage	V_0	V_1	V_2	V_3	Total
0	2,625				2,625
1	1,706				1,706
2	1,110				1,110
3	721	106			827
4	469	197			666
5	304	251			555
6	197	252	4		453
7	129	228	13		370
8	84	193	25		302
9	55	156	35		246
10	35	124	42	1	202
11	23	98	46	2	169
12	15	75	46	3	139
13	10	55	43	5	113
14	6	41	39	7	93

$$V_1(6) = \frac{721 \times 403 + 1,110 \times 489 + 1,706 \times 467 + 2,625 \times 338}{10,000} = 252$$

and

$$V_2(8) = \frac{251 \times 403 + 197 \times 489 + 106 \times 467}{10,000} = 25.$$

CALCULATIONS WITH DIFFERENT VALUES OF v

Once calculations have been made for one value v, those for other values are greatly simplified. Let us take another value v' and designate by V'_0, V'_1, V'_2, ... the corresponding V conceptions.

V_0 and V'_0 may be deduced from the conceptions (A and V combined) by multiplying the number of conceptions by v for V_0, and v' for V'_0. Hence, we have:

$$\frac{V'_0}{V_0} = \frac{v'}{v}. \tag{A11}$$

The series V_1 is obtained from the series V_0 by a number of operations of which only one, the product by $1 - v$, depends on v. Since V_0 follows from the series of conceptions from one multiplication by v one has:

$$\frac{V'_1}{V_1} = \frac{v'(1-v')}{v(1-v)} .$$ (A12)

Since we pass from V_1 to V_2 by operations of which only one, the product by $1-v$, depends on v, one has:

$$\frac{V'_2}{V_2} = \frac{v'(1-v')^2}{v(1-v)^2}$$ (A13)

and so on.

CHANGE IN MORTALITY
AFTER THE FIRST INTRA-UTERINE DEATH

The preceding calculations were made on the assumption that the incidence of intra-uterine mortality is constant. Let us now consider the case where the risk would change after the first death.

Let v_0 be the probability that the first conception ends in a live birth and v_1 the analogous probability for conceptions of order 2 and above that were preceded by an A conception.

In Eq. (A4), the expression for the number of deaths d, of month j, $\frac{1-v}{v}$ is replaced by $\frac{1-v_0}{v_0}$; but in the numbers a_0, a_1, a_2, ... (as in footnote 18) v is replaced by v_1. Hence, the coefficient a to be utilized in this case in order to pass from V_0 to V_1 is equal to:

$$\alpha_i = \frac{1-v_0}{v_0} \times v_1 \gamma_i$$ (A14)

while in the preceding case it was $(1-v)\gamma$ as given in (A10).

Since we assume that mortality changes only after the first intra-uterine death, the coefficient a which allows us to pass from V_1 to V_2, from V_2 to V_3 is $(1-v_1)\,\gamma$, that is to say it takes the same form as when mortality does not change, but with v_1 substituting for v.

Let us now use these results to calculate V'_0, V'_1, V'_2 ... (corresponding to the two probabilities v_0 and v_1) from the V_0, V_1, V_2 ... already calculated, corresponding to the same fecundability and the constant probability v. One has, for the same reasons as in the preceding section:

$$\frac{V'_0}{V_0} = \frac{v_0}{v} .$$ (A15)

The series V_1 follows from V_0 by a number of operations of which only the product involving $1 - v$ depends on v; in the passage from V'_0 to V'_1, the operation that depends on intra-uterine mortality is the product by $\dfrac{1-v_0}{v_0} v_1$. It follows that:

$$\frac{V'_1}{V_1} = \frac{\dfrac{1-v_0}{v_0} v_1 V'_0}{(1-v) V_0} = \frac{(1-v_0) v_1}{(1-v) v}. \tag{A16}$$

Since one passes respectively from V_1 to V_2 or from V'_1 to V'_2 by operations of which only one, the product by $1 - v$ or by $1 - v_1$, depends on the intra-uterine mortality, one has:

$$\frac{V'_2}{V_2} = \frac{1-v_1}{1-v} \cdot \frac{V'_1}{V_1} = \frac{(1-v_0) v_1(1-v_1)}{(1-v)^2 v}. \tag{A17}$$

We simplify the calculations by taking v equal to v_0. One then has:

$$V'_0 = V_0$$

$$V'_1 = \frac{v_1}{v_0} V_1$$

$$V'_2 = \frac{v_1(1-v_1)}{v_0(1-v_0)} V_2$$

$$V'_3 = \frac{v_1(1-v_1)^2}{v_0(1-v_0)^2} V_3. \tag{A18}$$

HETEROGENEOUS GROUPS

The situation is much more complicated for heterogeneous groups: fecundability is not distributed in the same way, for example, among women who conceived the first month as among those who conceived the second. Consequently, the distribution of conceptions after month 3 in the case of women who have had an A conception during month 0 followed by an intra-uterine death in month one, is not the same as the distribution of conceptions after month 4 among women that had an A conception in month 0 or 1, followed by an intra-uterine death in month 2. Hence, one can study heterogeneous groups only by combining the results obtained for homogeneous groups.

Appendix 3

PEARSON TYPE I DISTRIBUTION

We have no direct observations on the distribution of fecundability in a population. One can, however, assume that it is one of the general types studied by Pearson. Since fecundability can range between 0 and 1, it is natural to think that its distribution may be of type I, i.e., that the probability density of fecundability p is of the form:

$$h(p) = A p^{a-1} (1-p)^{b-1} \qquad \text{(A19)}$$

with:

$$A = \frac{\Gamma(a+b)}{\Gamma(a)\,\Gamma(b)}$$

For fixed p, the probability of still not having conceived at the beginning of month n is $(1-p)^n$; the corresponding probability of conceiving in the course of this month is $[p(1-p)^n$ —L.H.]. For all the women, the probability of not having conceived in month n is equal to:

$$A \int_0^1 p^{a-1} (1-p)^{b+n-1}\, dp = A\,\frac{\Gamma(a)\,\Gamma(b+n)}{\Gamma(a+b+n)}\,, \qquad \text{(A20)}$$

and the probability of conceiving in month n is:

$$c_n = A \int_0^1 p^{a} (1-p)^{b+n-1}\, dp = \frac{A\,\Gamma(a+1)\,\Gamma(b+n)}{\Gamma(a+b+n+1)}. \qquad \text{(A21)}$$

One therefore has for the rate q_n:

$$q_n = \frac{\Gamma(a+1)}{\Gamma(a)} \cdot \frac{\Gamma(a+b+n)}{\Gamma(a+b+n+1)} = \frac{a}{a+b+n}. \qquad \text{(A22)}$$

The inverse of q_n is a linear function of n.

The ratio r_n of the number of conceptions of month n to those of month $n-1$ is equal to:

$$r_n = \frac{\Gamma(a+1)\,\Gamma(b+n)}{\Gamma(a+b+n+1)} \cdot \frac{\Gamma(a+b+n)}{\Gamma(a+1)\,\Gamma(b+n-1)} = \frac{b+n-1}{a+b+n} \qquad \text{(A23)}$$

from which:

$$1 - r_n = \frac{a+1}{a+b+n} \qquad \text{(A24)}$$

and

$$\frac{1 - r_n}{q_n} = \frac{a + 1}{a}. \qquad (A25)$$

The probability of conceiving in month 0 is equal to the mean value of p:

$$c_0 = A \int_0^1 p \cdot p^{a-1} (1-p)^{b-1} \, dp = \frac{a}{a+b}. \qquad (A26)$$

One can determine the values for subsequent months with the help of the ratio r_n. The probability of conceiving in month n can be obtained by multiplying the probability for month $n - 1$ by r_n. Thus, one has for month 1:

$$c_1 = c_0 \times r_1 = \frac{a}{a+b} \times r_1 = \frac{a}{a+b} \times \frac{b}{a+b+1}. \qquad (A27)$$

Appendix 4

DISTRIBUTION OF FECUNDABILITY

One may construct heterogeneous groups *a priori*. The simplest way is to make them up from two homogeneous subgroups; it is, however, unlikely that real groups are so simple. Probably the whole gamut of possible values is represented and certain values are more common than others. One tends to assume, because it is a common situation, that the distribution is unimodal. As stated in Appendix 3, a Pearson type I distribution is convenient and gives a good approximation to unimodal distributions that are encountered in reality, for a variable that, like fecundability, ranges between 0 and 1. We will then attempt to construct a heterogeneous group where fecundabilities are distributed almost like those in a Pearson type I distribution. However, to determine the parameters of this distribution it is necessary to have some idea of the dispersion of fecundability.

Consider a heterogeneous group with a mean fecundability $\bar{p}$ and with a mean intra-uterine mortality $(1 - v)$. The probability of V conceptions is equal to $v\bar{p}$ for the first month and to $v\bar{p} - v\bar{p}^2 (1 + c^2)$ for the second month, where c is the coefficient of variation of fecundability.[19] The ratio r_1 of the probability of a V conception in the second month to that the first month is then equal to:

$$r_1 = 1 - \bar{p}(1 + c^2). \tag{A28}$$

One therefore has:

$$1 - r_1 = \bar{p}(1 + c^2),$$

and

$$\frac{1 - r_1}{q_0} = \frac{\bar{p}(1 + c^2)}{v\bar{p}} = \frac{1 + c^2}{v}. \tag{A29}$$

Because of fluctuations caused by the timing of marriage in the menstrual cycle, this formula is not applicable to crude data. Moreover, in differences such as are being used here, the effects of chance fluctuations are magnified. We will, therefore, try to evaluate the coefficient of variation from adjusted values of the fertility rates of the first two months. Thus, we obtain for $\frac{1 + c^2}{v}$, the value 1.75 from the historical data, and 1.37 from the modern data.

Since the modern data are derived from a selected group, their intra-uterine mortality is, certainly, lower than in the combined historical data. For the latter, one can expect an intra-uterine mortality of the order of 15 to 20 percent,[20] which would give values between 0.40 and 0.49 for c^2. For the modern group one would have $c^2 = 0.23$ only with an intra-uterine mortality of 10 percent. The spread between the two estimates is large; lacking other data we have taken an intermediate value, i.e. $c^2 \approx 0.3$. We note before continuing, that these results, though very imprecise, indicate that real groups are quite heterogeneous in fecundability.

---

[19] The probability of a V conception in the second month is equal to:

$$v \, E \, p(1 - p) = v\bar{p} - v \, E \, p^2 = v\bar{p} - v\bar{p}^2 \, (1 + c^2)$$

$$= v\bar{p} - v\bar{p}^2 \left(\frac{\sigma^2 + \bar{p}^2}{\bar{p}^2} \right).$$

[20] Where intra-uterine mortality depends on pregnancy order, if one assumes 25 percent for all pregnancies, one would have 17 percent for first pregnancies according to the results published in S. Shapiro et al. [1].

TABLE A3
DISTRIBUTION A OF FECUNDABILITY

Fecundability	Frequency
0.05	0.1
0.15	0.2
0.25	0.2
0.35	0.2
0.45	0.1
0.55	0.1
0.65	0.1

In practice, we have replaced the continuous distribution by a discrete distribution, which must therefore be simpler. After some trials, we chose Distribution A in Table A3, which is quite close to a Type I Pearson distribution. It has a mean of 0.320 and $c^2 = 0.313$.

To see how the results change if another distribution is used we also tried Distribution B, which includes only 6 fecundabilities: 0.05, 0.15, 0.25, 0.35, 0.45 and 0.55, each with the same frequency; the mean is 0.300 and $c^2 = 0.323$.

Appendix 5

DISPERSION OF INTRA-UTERINE MORTALITY

Let us assume that every woman has a constant risk of intra-uterine mortality at least for some years. Then, observed differences in risk for women whose preceding pregnancies ended in a spontaneous abortion as opposed to the risk for those who had a live birth are due to the unequal risks of spontaneous abortion among different women.

Let v be the probability that a conception ends in a live birth and $h(v)$ be the probability density of v. Consider two consecutive pregnancies. The probability that the first pregnancy ends in a live birth is equal to:

$$\int_0^1 vh(v)\,dv = \bar{v} \qquad (A30)$$

where $\bar{v}$ is the mean value of v. The probability that it ends in a spontaneous abortion is $1 - \bar{v}$.

If c^2 is the squared coefficient of variation of v, the probability that the second pregnancy ends in a spontaneous abortion, given that the first terminated in a live birth, is equal to:[21]

$$\alpha_1 = \frac{\int_0^1 (1-v)\, vh(v)\, dv}{\int_0^1 vh(v)\, dv} = 1 - \bar{v} - \bar{v}c^2. \qquad (A31)$$

If the first pregnancy terminated in a spontaneous abortion, the probability of an abortion at the second pregnancy is equal to:

$$\alpha_2 = \frac{\int_0^1 (1-v)^2\, h(v)\, dv}{\int_0^1 (1-v)\, h(v)\, dv} = (1 - \bar{v}) + \frac{\bar{v}^2\, c^2}{1 - \bar{v}}. \qquad (A32)$$

We have:

$$\alpha_2 - \alpha_1 = c^2 \left(\frac{\bar{v}^2}{1 - \bar{v}} + \bar{v} \right) = c^2 \frac{\bar{v}}{1 - \bar{v}}, \qquad (A33)$$

and

$$1 - \bar{v} = \frac{\alpha_1}{1 + \alpha_1 - \alpha_2}. \qquad (A34)$$

In the previously cited report of Shapiro et al., one finds the following values of a_1 and a_2 per 1000 pregnancies of orders 2 and 3:

	a_2 per 1,000	a_1
Order 2	156	92
Order 3	216	112

which gives the following values of $\bar{v}$ and c^2:

	$\bar{v}$ per 1,000	c_2
Order 2	902	0.007
Order 3	875	0.015

These observations were not analyzed as were those from Kauai, by the life table method; the probability of intra-uterine

---

[21] [The functions denoted by the symbols α_i used here bear no relation to those denoted by the same symbols in Eq. (A8).]

TABLE A4
HYPOTHETICAL DISTRIBUTION OF PROBABILITY
OF INTRA-UTERINE SURVIVAL (v)

v	Weight	v	Weight
0.65	0.1	0.85	0.2
0.70	0.1	0.90	0.2
0.75	0.1	0.95	0.1
0.80	0.2		

mortality was, consequently, greatly underestimated. One may, on the other hand, accept, at least as an order of magnitude, the values for the coefficient of variation.

If one assumes, as was done for fecundability, that v, which can assume values from 0 to 1, has approximately a Pearson Type I distribution, we would know this distribution from $\bar{v}$ and c^2. For first conceptions, $\bar{v}$ should be of the order of 80 percent to 85 percent, which a Pearson curve with the parameter a about five times the parameter b would fit $\left(\text{since } \bar{v} = \dfrac{a}{a+b} \right).$

Accordingly, we started, for convenience, with a distribution corresponding to $a = 10$, $b = 2$; c^2 is equal to 0.015. As in the case of fecundability, we then replaced this distribution by a simpler distribution shown in Table A4. This distribution has its mean $\bar{v} = 0.815$ with $c^2 = 0.012$.

CHAPTER SIX

An Attempt to Calculate the Effectiveness of Contraception*

EDITORS' SUMMARY

Under several assumptions regarding the distribution of fecundability in a population using contraceptives, this paper (published in 1968) studies the relation between the mean value of fecundability and the value of what Henry calls the Improved Pearl Index. Henry concludes that in certain defined situations, the latter Index may be used to estimate mean fecundability.

*Originally printed in French as "Essai de calcul de l'efficacité de la contraception." *Population* 23, no. 2 (Mars-Avril 1968): 265-278.

CONTENTS

INTRODUCTION

Several years ago, *Population* published a historical review of methods of evaluating contraceptive effectiveness, difficulties met therein, and some results (Seklani [1]). As shown in detail below, the current situation is as follows. On the one hand, we have a correct definition of effectiveness; on the other hand, we have a series of numerical values of an index—which we, for convenience, call the Improved Pearl Index—that depends both on contraceptive effectiveness and on the distribution of fecundability during contraception, i.e. the residual fecundability of married women using contraceptives. To our knowledge, there has been little attempt to establish any relationship, even an approximate one, between the Improved Pearl Index and effectiveness, doubtless because of our ignorance of the distribution of residual fecundability among women.

In this article we propose to examine how such a distribution affects the relation in question and, if necessary, how one can use the Improved Pearl Index to estimate the value, or the order of magnitude, of effectiveness.

SUMMARY OF NOTATION

$R_x, R(x)$	Discrete and continuous versions respectively of the Pearl Index calculated at month x of exposure to risk.
r	Residual fecundability (with the use of contraception).
$f(r)$	P.d.f. of r.
$\bar{r}$	Mean value of $f(r)$.
m_2 and m_3	Noncentral second and third moments of $f(r)$.

FAILURES AND EFFECTIVENESS

Although it seems most natural to consider that a contraceptive method is very effective if it results in only few failures, this natural idea leads nowhere: the risk of failure depends on the duration of contraceptive practice, which is known as the duration of exposure to risk. Table 1 shows the probability of failure (i.e. at least one undesired conception) according to the duration of exposure to risk, at a level of effectiveness that is often achieved currently (98 percent), giving a mean residual fecundability of 0.005.

TABLE 1

PROBABILITY OF FAILURE
BY DURATION OF EXPOSURE TO RISK

Duration of Exposure to Risk	Percent of Expected Failures
5 years	26
10 years	45
15 years	60
20 years	70

Since the probability of failure increases with the duration of exposure to risk, an index of effectiveness must be based on failures *per unit time.*

THE PEARL INDEX

It seems simple to satisfy this condition by relating undesired conceptions to the duration of exposure to risk. Following such reasoning, Raymond Pearl constructed the index which is given his name here (see Pearl's rate I in Chapter one). Instead of taking the month as the time unit, he took the century, but since the month, serving for the menstrual cycle, is retained as the unit of observation, the index, denoted by R, is calculated as follows:

$$R = \frac{\text{number of undesired conceptions} \times 1200}{\text{number of months of exposure to risk}}.$$

This index has been known as the conception rate or pregnancy rate; it appears under the latter name in the Multilingual Demographic Dictionary.

Currently it is known as the "failure rate" in English. One must not confuse this rate per unit time with the probability of failure, which was shown in Table 1 to mean something rather different.

CORRECT DEFINITION
OF EFFECTIVENESS

At the time when Pearl introduced the above index, C. Gini had already introduced the notion of fecundability. For a variety of reasons, however, this notion at first received little attention. It is only since the war that this important notion has been given its place among the accepted ideas of demography.

Fecundability is the probability that a married woman will conceive in the course of a menstrual cycle (in practice, the menstrual cycle is replaced by the month). Nothing prevents the application of this idea to cases where contraception is practiced, as well as where it is not practiced; it suffices to distinguish these cases by calling the latter *natural* fecundability and the former *residual* fecundability.

The ratio of residual fecundability to natural fecundability would be a good index of effectiveness. It would, however, have the disadvantage of decreasing as effectiveness increases; therefore we prefer its complement. Thus, an effectiveness of 98 percent, mentioned above, means that residual fecundability is equal to

TABLE 2
PEARL INDEX (R) FOR VARIOUS PERIODS OF OBSERVATION
(FROM DATA IN WESTOFF ET AL.)

Observation Period	R
1 month	42.4
6 months or less	37.1
12 months or less	35.7
18 months or less	30.8
24 months or less	29.4
36 months or less	27.3
48 months or less	26.2

[Note: The exposure time of a woman who had been married for 16 months, for example, and had never conceived is counted in all the calculations up to 12 months or less, but not in the subsequent calculations. A woman who conceived 16 months after marriage contributes 1 month of exposure time to the first row, 6 months to the second, 12 months to the third and thereafter she counts as one pregnancy and 16 months of exposure.]

2 percent of natural fecundability.[1] One could also define an average effectiveness as the ratio of the mean residual fecundability to the mean natural fecundability. In practice, we are almost always interested in the average effectiveness of a contraceptive method or of a number of such methods.

DEFECTS OF THE PEARL INDEX

The Pearl Index (R), which gives the number of undesired conceptions per unit time, seems at first glance to be appropriate. It is, however, not at all suitable.

Observed groups of contracepting couples are heterogeneous with respect both to natural fecundability and to contraceptive effectiveness. Hence they are even more heterogeneous with respect to residual fecundability. Because of this heterogeneity, women with the highest residual fecundability conceive and leave observation earlier and, consequently, the composition of the group changes constantly, with a progressive decrease in the mean residual fecundability of the group. The Pearl Index therefore varies with the duration of observation, as illustrated by the series of values, in Table 2, taken from a survey in the United States in 1957 and 1960 (Westoff [2]).

[1] This definition of effectiveness was introduced by Potter [1] in 1960; the idea was already present in an article of Tietze [1].

Thus, a specified method can appear more or less effective according to whether observations were continued for a longer or shorter period. It follows that comparisons between values of R must be based on observation periods of the same duration, a condition that eliminates almost all published series of R indices because the duration of the observation period has not been specified.[2]

IMPROVEMENT OF THE PEARL INDEX

Surveys in depth that provide data on contraceptive practice necessarily include rather few individuals. If the periods of observation were limited to very short durations, as is suggested by theoretical considerations, much information would be lost. In addition, the onset of exposure to risk is poorly defined after a delivery, partly because of the difficulty of obtaining sufficiently precise information on the duration of amenorrhea, and also, even more important, because there is probably an increased incidence of anovular cycles immediately following postpartum amenorrhea.

A very long period of observation has the disadvantage either of complicating the calculations if one includes couples who deliberately interrupt contraception in order to conceive before the end of the observation period, or of losing information if these couples are eliminated because of this complication.

Hence an intermediate period of observation seems desirable. For example, the American survey already cited (Westoff [2]), used a period of 12 months. It is this index that we call the Improved Pearl Index, and which we denote by the symbol R_{12} in what follows.

THE RELATION BETWEEN THE IMPROVED PEARL INDEX AND THE MEAN RESIDUAL [FECUNDABILITY —L.H.]

As shown in the Appendix, the Improved Pearl Index, R_{12}, is connected to the mean residual fecundability, $\bar{r}$, by a relationship

---

[2] This effect of the length of the observation period was brought out by Potter [1].

TABLE 3

MEAN AND STANDARD DEVIATION OF FOUR
POSSIBLE DISTRIBUTIONS OF RESIDUAL FECUNDABILITY

Distribution Number	Mean Fecundability	Standard Deviation
1	0.0380	0.0536
2	0.0424	0.0650
3	0.0400	0.0821
4	0.0609	0.1134

that includes all the moments of the residual fecundability. It is therefore impossible, in principle, to calculate $\bar{r}$ from R_{12} unless this distribution is known. The survey already cited has provided at least an approximate idea of this distribution. (Potter [2]). A Pearson Type III distribution was assumed *a priori* and the parameters were estimated so that the expected proportions of women conceiving at specified durations of marriage, according to this distribution, correspond with observed values among contracepting couples.

Four possible distributions were used, of which the second was considered to be the most suitable. Their means and standard deviations are shown in Table 3.

[For the data in Table 3, values of the parameters (a and k) of corresponding Pearson Type III distributions were estimated as described in the Appendix and shown in Table A1.

With the use of Eq. (A16), values of R_{12} were calculated for each distribution. Table 4 shows these values] $\bar{r}$, R_{12} and the ratio R_{12}/R_1, where R_1 denotes the Pearl Index calculated at an observation period of one month. Since $R_1 = 1,200\ \bar{r}$, it follows from Table 4 that $R_{12}/1,200$ ranges from about one-half to three-fourths of the mean residual fecundability, the most plausible value being about two-thirds.

The same survey also showed that contraceptive effectiveness increases with increasing parity, and that this increase is particularly marked when the number of births reaches the number of children desired (Westoff et al. [2]).

The distributions in Table 3 correspond to the situation at the beginning of marriage and consequently to a moderate mean effectiveness. To study further the relations between R_{12} and $\bar{r}$ it is necessary to see what would be the case for much smaller values of $\bar{r}$.

TABLE 4

MEAN RESIDUAL FECUNDABILITY, $\bar{r}$,
IMPROVED PEARL INDEX, R_{12}, AND RATIO R_{12}/R_1
USING THE FOUR POSSIBLE DISTRIBUTIONS

Distribution	$\bar{r}$	R_{12}	R_{12}/R_1 (Percent)
1	0.0380	32.9	72
2	0.0424	34.3	67.5
3	0.0490	35.6	60.5
4	0.0609	37.8	52

Undoubtedly, effectiveness improves more for couples with low initial effectiveness than for others. A distribution based on an assumption that residual [fecundability —L.H.] decreases in the same proportion for all couples, would be more dispersed than distributions with the same mean obtained by assuming that residual fecundability decreases relatively more when it was higher at the beginning of marriage. Hence, the first assumption leads to a maximum estimate of the discrepancy between R_{12} and R_1.

Distributions of r were postulated, with means that were one-tenth, one-fifth, or one-half of each of the values in Table 4, and under two assumptions regarding the variance: (a) assuming that all women had an identical relative decrease in effective fecundability, and (b) a variance of zero. Table 5 shows the results —the lower value of R_{12} in each case corresponds to the first assumption and $R_1 = R_{12}$ corresponds to the second.

Figure 1, which illustrates Tables 4 and 5, shows a close relation between R_{12} and $\bar{r}$ when R_{12} is low. Also, considering the variations in these two quantities, the relation between the two is still

TABLE 5

EXTREME VALUES OF IMPROVED PEAL INDEX, R_{12},
FOR VARIOUS VALUES
OF THE MEAN RESIDUAL FECUNDABILITY, $\bar{r}$

$\bar{r}$	R_{12}		$\bar{r}$	R_{12}	
	Minimum	Maximum		Minimum	Maximum
0.0038	4.4	4.5	0.0098	10.2	11.8
0.0042	4.8	5.0	0.0122	11.9	14.6
0.0049	5.5	5.9	0.0190	19.0	22.8
0.0061	6.7	7.5	0.0212	20.2	25.4
0.0076	8.4	9.1	0.0245	21.6	29.4
0.0085	9.1	10.2	0.0305	24.0	36.6

useful for moderate values. At higher values of R_{12}, any one value of R_{12} corresponds to a large range of values of $\bar{r}$. From the results in Table 4, one may nevertheless replace the region of these points (R_{12}, 1,000 $\bar{r}$) by the zone marked in dots, this substitution meaning only that the points (R_{12}, 1,000 $\bar{r}$) would be found more frequently in this zone than outside of it.

In any case, when R_{12} is greater than about 35, it corresponds poorly with $\bar{r}$ because $\bar{r}$ apparently increases rapidly while R_{12} increases only at a moderate rate.

RELATIONS BETWEEN R_{12} AND EFFECTIVENESS

The mean natural fecundability of all newlyweds certainly lies between 0.25 and 0.35, and probably, for women married between the ages of 20 and 30, it is approximately 0.30.

In Figure 1, we have shown values of residual fecundability corresponding to an effectiveness of 90, 95, 98, and 99 percent. In the lower part of the graph, it may be seen that the points (R_{12}, 1,000 $\bar{r}$) corresponding to each value of effectiveness are in a very narrow band (hatched). In the upper part of the graph, the range is too indefinite and we have simply indicated the extreme points, in the dotted area, of the limits of the interval corresponding to an effectiveness of 90 percent. From this graph, an approximate relation between the improved Pearl Index and the effectiveness can be shown as in Table 6.[3]

TABLE 6

APPROXIMATE RELATION BETWEEN IMPROVED PEARL INDEX
AND EFFECTIVENESS

R_{12}	Effectiveness (Percent)
1.5 to 2	99.5
3 to 4	99
6 to 8	98
12 to 21	95
About 30	90

[3] C. Tietze [1] gives a table showing an analogous correspondence between effectiveness and R_{12}; but in his table R_{12} is calculated according to a model, while we have tried to establish a relation between observed values of R_{12} and average effectiveness.

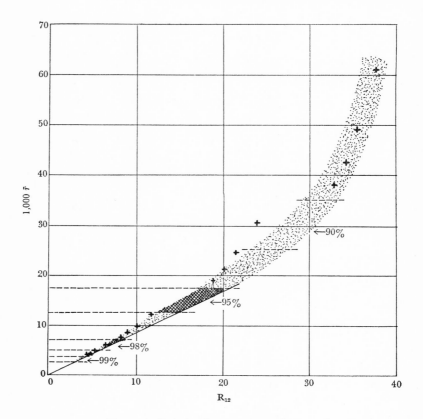

Figure 1. Relation between R_{12} and $\bar{r}$.

Until now, we have considered only observations made at the beginning of marriage. In the case of other observations, there is an additional difficulty: the beginning of the period of exposure to risk following a delivery is poorly defined. If the duration of nonsusceptibility is underestimated, effectiveness is credited with what is due only to a delay in the resumption of ovulation or of sexual relations; if this duration is overestimated, effectiveness is also overestimated, since couples with the highest residual [fecundability —L.H.] have already left observation in a larger proportion than others, following an unplanned conception.

In the survey already cited, the onset of exposure to risk was

TABLE 7

VALUES OF R BETWEEN MARRIAGE
AND THE FIRST CONCEPTION (1), BETWEEN THE FIRST BIRTH
AND THE NEXT CONCEPTION (2), AND THE CORRESPONDING RATIO (3)
BY PERIODS OF OBSERVATION (DATA FROM WESTOFF ET AL.)

Duration of Observation Period	Beginning from Marriage (1)	After 1st Birth (2)	Ratio (3) = (2)/(1)
1 month	42.4	14.5	0.34
6 months or less	37.1	25.1	0.68
12 months or less	35.7	24.7	0.69
18 months or less	30.8	23.8	0.77
24 months or less	29.4	22.3	0.76
36 months or less	27.3	20.8	0.76
48 months or less	26.2	19.9	0.76

placed at one month following delivery. Table 7 shows the values of R in the interval between the first birth and the following conception, according to the duration of observation. We recall the corresponding values of R at the beginning of marriage and calculate the ratio of the two.

Clearly, at one month after delivery the risk of an undesired conception is still, for at least one month, considerably below normal. The inclusion of the nonsusceptible period, for certain women, in the total duration of exposure to risk also affects estimated values of R other than R_1, but it seems to have scarcely any further effect beyond R_{12} and it lowers R_{12} only by about 10 percent below the value it ought to have. Considering the degree of imprecision that can be tolerated in the relation between R_{12} and $\bar{r}$, this discrepancy of 10 percent is negligible. One may then, in conclusion, consider that Table 6 is valid for all values of R_{12}, whether they relate to the interval between marriage and the first conception, the interval between the first birth and the second conception or to another interval.

EXAMPLE

The investigation previously cited showed that contraceptive effectiveness improves in the course of marriage even without any change in the method used, through the effects of increased care alone. The direct effect of motivation can be seen there: while motivation is relatively weak as long as it is a question only of

TABLE 8

PEARL INDEX, R_{12}, AND EFFECTIVENESS OF CONTRACEPTION
(IN PERCENT) FOR COUPLES WITH DIFFERENT NUMBERS
OF DESIRED CHILDREN (DATA FROM WESTOFF ET AL.)

Interval	Number of Children Desired—Pearl Index R_{12}			Number of Children Desired—Effectiveness		
	2	3	4 or more	2	3	4 or more
Marriage to 1st pregnancy	21.1	26.6	45.9	90–95	90–95	less than 90
1st to 2nd pregnancy	7.8	13.7	16.3	98	95	95
Since the 2nd live birth	2.6	16.5	13.4	99	95	95

deferring the first birth, it becomes stronger with respect to the spacing of births and very strong when, after the birth of the last desired child, the couple has really decided not to have any more.

Table 8 relates to couples that have used, from marriage to the time of the survey, one of the three most effective methods of the period (condom, diaphragm or coitus interruptus). At the left are shown values of R_{12}, and on the right those of the corresponding effectiveness.

For all couples who have practived any contraceptive method whatsoever in the three intervals, the average effectiveness is shown in Table 9.

The levels are generally lower than in Table 8, but here also effectiveness increases with interval order in a similar manner. The contraception of limitation (following the birth of the last desired child) is notably more effective than the contraception of spacing, itself more effective than the contraception of delay, designed simply to defer the first conception.[4]

These results have two very important aspects. They show first that the intensity of motivation is much more important than the particular contraceptive method used. From this fact, we understand much better why limitation should have been able to be very effective in relatively early times, since coitus interruptus can assure great effectiveness as long as motivation is sufficiently strong.

These results also show how an effectiveness that is relatively low when all intervals are considered may be found together

---

[4] This terminology is taken from A. Jacquard, [1].

TABLE 9
EFFECTIVENESS OF CONTRACEPTION (IN PERCENT)
FOR ALL COUPLES USING ANY CONTRACEPTIVE METHOD,
BY NUMBER OF CHILDREN DESIRED

Interval	Number of Children Desired		
	2	3	4 or more
Marriage to 1st pregnancy	90	less than 90	less than 90
1st to 2nd pregnancy	95	95	90
After the 2nd live2birth	99	95	between 90 and 95

with a relatively small proportion of couples that have more children than they desire. The latter proportion depends on the duration of exposure to risk following the last desired birth and on the effectiveness of the contraception *of limitation*, which is much greater than the overall effectiveness.

Appendix

Here we will attempt to calculate $R(x)$, where x is the time since the beginning of exposure to risk, as a function of the distribution of residual fecundability.

GENERAL CASE

Let r be the residual fecundability per unit of time. Then, $(1 - r)^x$ is the proportion of women of fecundability r who have not yet conceived at time x and $1 - (1 - r)^x$ is the proportion of women who have had an undesired conception. The total number of months of exposure to risk up to time x is therefore equal to:

$$\sum_{0}^{x-1} (1-r)^\xi = \frac{1}{r} [1 - (1-r)^x]. \tag{A1}$$

If $f(r)$ is the p.d.f. of r, it follows that:

$$R(x) = \frac{\int_0^1 [1 - (1-r)^x] f(r)\, dr}{\int_0^1 \frac{1}{r} [1 - (1-r)^x] f(r)\, dr} \times 1,200, \tag{A2}$$

which shows that $R(x)/1,200$ is the ratio of the total undesired conceptions from month 0 until month $x - 1$ inclusive, to the total exposure to risk. We will develop $(1 - r)^x$ as a series and introduce the noncentral moments $\bar{r}$, m_2, and m_3 of $f(r)$. Since r

is less than 1, usually considerably so, these moments are considerably less than 1 and decrease rapidly as the order of the moment increases.

If, in addition, x is not too large, one may write:

$$\frac{R(x)}{1,200} \approx \frac{\bar{r} - m_2 \dfrac{(x-1)}{2} + m_3 \dfrac{(x-1)(x-2)}{6}}{1 - \bar{r} \dfrac{(x-1)}{2} + m_2 \dfrac{(x-1)(x-2)}{6}} \cdot \qquad \text{(A3)}$$

Putting:

$$x - 1 = u \qquad \text{and } (x-1)(x-2) = v^2, \qquad \text{(A4)}$$

Eq. (A3) may be written as:

$$\frac{R(x)}{1,200} \approx \bar{r} \cdot \frac{1 - \dfrac{m_2}{\bar{r}} \dfrac{u}{2} + \dfrac{m_3}{\bar{r}} \dfrac{v^2}{6}}{1 - \bar{r} \dfrac{u}{2} + m_2 \dfrac{v^2}{6}} \cdot \qquad \text{(A5)}$$

The coefficient of $\bar{r}$, of the form $\left(\dfrac{1-a}{1-b}\right)$, may be written as: $(1-a)(1+b+b^2+\ldots)$ or, keeping terms of order 1 and 2 only, $1 + b - a + b(b-a)$. Hence, Eq. (A5) to terms in u^2 and v^2, is equal to:

$$\frac{R(x)}{1,200} \approx \bar{r} \left[1 + \left(\bar{r} - \frac{m_2}{\bar{r}}\right)\frac{u}{2} + \left(\frac{m_3}{\bar{r}} - m_2\right)\frac{v^2}{6} + \bar{r}\left(\bar{r} - \frac{m_2}{\bar{r}}\right)\frac{u^2}{4} \right]$$
$$\text{(A6)}$$

or, if σ^2 is the variance of r,

$$\frac{R(x)}{1,200} \approx \bar{r} \left[1 - \sigma^2 \frac{u}{2\bar{r}} + \left(\frac{m_3}{\bar{r}} - m_2\right)\frac{v^2}{6} - \sigma^2 \frac{u^2}{4} \right]. \qquad \text{(A7)}$$

But since $v^2 = u^2 - u$, we have:

$$\frac{R(x)}{1,200} \approx \bar{r} \cdot \{1 - \frac{u}{6\bar{r}}[3\sigma^2 + m_3 - \bar{r}m_2] + \frac{u^2}{12\bar{r}}[2m_3 - 2\bar{r}m_2 - 3\bar{r}\sigma^2]\}. \qquad \text{(A8)}$$

But if μ_3 is the third central moment, i.e.

$$\mu_3 = m_2 - 3\bar{r}m_2 + 2\bar{r}^3 = m_3 - \bar{r}m_2 - 2\bar{r}\sigma^2,$$

we have:

$$\frac{R(x)}{1,200} \approx \bar{r} \{1 - \frac{u}{6\bar{r}}[3\sigma^2 + \mu_3 + 2\bar{r}\sigma^2] + \frac{u^2}{12\bar{r}}[2\mu_3 + \bar{r}\sigma^2]\}. \qquad \text{(A9)}$$

When $u\bar{r}$ is sufficiently small, the principal term on the right hand side of Eq. (A9) is $1 - \dfrac{u}{2\bar{r}}\sigma^2$ and the discrepancy between $R(x)$ and $\bar{r}$ decreases as the variance of r decreases.

[The results in Eqs. (A3) to (A9) were not used for the numerical examples, which were calculated on the assumptions considered below.]

CASE WHERE $f(r)$ IS A PEARSON TYPE III DISTRIBUTION

A Pearson Type III distribution can be treated only in the continuous case, as was done in the article cited (Potter [2]).[5] In this case, we have:

$$R(x) = \frac{\int_0^\infty (1 - e^{-rx}) f(r) \, dr}{\int_0^\infty \frac{1}{r} (1 - e^{-rx}) f(r) \, dr} \times 1,200, \tag{A10}$$

since the total duration of exposure to risk from time 0 up to time x is equal to:

$$\int_0^x e^{-r\xi} \, d\xi = \frac{1}{r} (1 - e^{-rx}). \tag{A11}$$

In addition,

$$f(r) = \frac{a^k}{\Gamma(k)} e^{-ar} r^{k-1}. \tag{A12}$$

[A Pearson Type III distribution as defined in Eq. (A12) has mean $m = k/a$ and variance $s^2 = k/a^2$. Hence if the mean (m) and variance (s^2) of a sample are known, a and k may be estimated as $\hat{a} = \dfrac{m}{s^2}$ and $\hat{k} = \hat{a}m$.] The numerator and the denominator of $R(x)$ in Eq. (A10) can each be presented in the form:

$$A \int_0^\infty (1 - e^{-rx}) e^{-ar} r^{h-1} \, dr, \tag{A13}$$

where A is equal to $\dfrac{a^k}{\Gamma(k)}$ and h is equal to k in the numerator and to $k - 1$ in the denominator. After integrating by parts, the integral in Eq. (A13) becomes:

---

[5] In fact, the distribution was fitted successively to the cumulative conceptions from 0 to b and from b to 24, where b was put equal to 3, 6, 9, and 12 months, in turn.

$$\left[\frac{1}{h}r^h(1 - e^{-rx})\,e^{-ar}\right]_0^\infty + \frac{1}{h}\int_0^\infty r^h[(a + x)\,e^{-r(a + x)} - ae^{-ar}]\,dr$$

$$(A14)$$

and reduces to the second term since the first term is zero.

In addition, we have

$$\int_0^\infty r^h(a + x)\,e^{-r(a + x)}\,dr = \frac{1}{(a + x)^h}\int_0^\infty u^h\,e^{-u}\,du = \frac{\Gamma(h + 1)}{(a + x)^h},$$

and

$$\int_0^\infty r^h\,a\,e^{-ar}\,dr = \frac{\Gamma(h + 1)}{a^h},\qquad (A15)$$

which gives:[6]

$$\frac{R(x)}{1,200} = \frac{k - 1}{k}\cdot\frac{\Gamma(k + 1)}{\Gamma(k)}\cdot\frac{\dfrac{1}{(a + x)^k} - \dfrac{1}{a^k}}{\dfrac{1}{(a + x)^{k-1}} - \dfrac{1}{a^{k-1}}}$$

$$= \frac{k - 1}{a}\cdot\frac{1 - \left(\dfrac{a}{a + x}\right)^k}{1 - \left(\dfrac{a}{a + x}\right)^{k-1}}.\qquad (A16)$$

The values of a and of k from the article by Potter et al. [2] cited in the text, are:

TABLE 1A

Mean Value of r	a	k
0.0380	13.22	0.502
0.0424	10.03	0.425
0.0490	7.27	0.356
0.0609	4.73	0.288

[If a new distribution is defined with $\bar{r}_1 = \dfrac{\bar{r}}{10}$ and $s_1^2 = \dfrac{s^2}{100}$, then $a_1 = 10a$ and $k_1 = k$. This result was used to derive the values presented in Table 5.]

---

[6] The difference between the values of $R(x)$ in the continuous case and in the discrete case, which is utilized in practice, is negligible. For the same number of conceptions in the numerator, the denominator in the discrete case contains one-half month more for women who have conceived. In other words for 30/1,200 in the continuous case, one has 30/1,215 in the discrete case.

References

Brass [1], William, "The distribution of births in human populations." *Population Studies* 12, no. 1 (July 1958): 51–72.

Dandekar [1], Kumudini, "Intervals between confinements." *Eugenics Quarterly* 6, no. 3 (September 1958): 180–186.

Dandekar [2], Kumudini, "Analysis of birth intervals of a set of Indian women." *Eugenics Quarterly* 10, no. 2 (June 1963): 73–78.

French [1], F. E., and J. M. Bierman, "Probabilities of fetal mortality." *Public Health Reports* 77, no. 10 (October 1962): 835–847.

Ganiage [1], Jean, *La population européenne de Tunis au milieu du XIXè siècle.* Paris: Presses Universitaires de France, 1960.

Ganiage [2], Jean, *Trois villages d'Ile-de-France. Etude démographique.* Paris: Presses Universitaires de France, Travaux et Documents de l'Institut National d'Etudes Démographiques, Cahier no. 40, 1963. P. 148.

Gautier [1], Etienne, and Louis Henry. *"La population de Crulai, paroisse normande."* Paris: Presses Universitaires de France, Travaux et Documents de l'Institut National d'Etudes Démographiques, Cahier no. 33, 1958. P. 272.

Gini [1], Corrado. Premières recherches sur la fécondabilité de la femme. Toronto: *Proceedings of the International Mathematics Congress,* 1924. P. 889–892.

Henripin, [1], Jacques. *La population canadienne au début du XVIIIè siècle. Nuptialité, fécondité, mortalité infantile.* Paris: Presses Universitaires de France, Travaux et Documents de l'Institut National d'Etudes Démographiques, Cahier no. 22, 1954. P. 129.

Henry [1], Louis. *Fécondité des mariages; nouvelle méthode de mesure.* Paris: Presses Universitares de France, Travaux et Documents de l'Institut National d'Etudes Démographiques, Cahier no. 16, 1953. P. 180.

Henry [2], Louis "Fondements théoriques des mesures de la fécondité naturelle." *Revue de l'Institut International de Statistique* 21, no. 3 (1953): 135–151.

Henry [3], Louis. *Anciennes familles genevoises. Etude démographique XVI–XXè siècles.* Paris: Presses Universitaires de France, Travaux et Documents de l'Institut National d'Etudes Démographiques, Cahier no. 26, 1956, P. 234.

Henry [4], Louis, "Caractéristiques démographiques des pays sous-développés" dans *Le Tiers Monde. Sous-développement et développment.* Ouvrage réalisé sous la direction de Georges Balandier. Paris: Presses Universitaires de France, Travaux et Documents de l'Institut National d'Etudes Démographiques, Cahier no. 27, 1956. P. 392.

Henry [5], Louis, "Fécondité et famille. Modèles mathématiques I." *Population* 12, no. 3 (July–September 1957): 413–333.

Henry [6], Louis, "Fécondité et famille. Modèles mathématiques II. Partie théorique." *Population* 16, no. 1 (January–February 1961): 27–48.

Henry [7], Louis, "Fécondité et famille. Modèles mathématiques II. Applications numériques." *Population* 16, no. 2 (March–April 1961): 261–282.

HENRY [8], LOUIS, "La fécondité naturelle. Observations-Théorie-Résultats." *Population* 16, no. 4 (October–December 1961): 625-636.

HENRY [9], LOUIS "Mesure du temps mort en fécondité naturelle." *Population* 19, no. 3 (June–July 1964): 485–514.

HENRY [10], LOUIS, "Mortalité intra-utérine et fécondabilité." *Population* 19, no. 5 (October–December 1964): 899–940.

HENRY [11], LOUIS, "Essai de calcul de l'efficacité de la contraception." *Population* 23, no. 2 (March–April 1968): 265–278.

HOUDAILLE [1], JACQUES, "Un village du Morvan: Saint-Agnan." *Population* 16, no. 2 (October–December 1961): 301–312.

JACQUARD [1],A., "La reproduction humaine en régime malthusien. Un modèle de simulation par la méthode de Monte-Carlo." *Population* 22, no. 5 (September–October 1967): 897–920.

OKASAKI [1], AYANORI. *Fertility of the Farming Population in Japan.* Tokyo: Research Institute of Population Problems, 1951.

PEARL [1], RAYMOND. *The Natural History of Population.* London: Oxford University Press, H. Milford, 1939. p. 416.

POTTER [1], R. G., "Length of observation period as affecting the contraceptive failure rate." *The Milbank Memorial Fund Quarterly* 38, no. 2 (April 1960): 140-152.

POTTER [2], R. G., P. C. SAGI, and C. F. WESTOFF, "Improvement of contraception during the course of marriage." *Population Studies* 16, no. 2 (November 1962): 160–174.

POTTER [3], R. G., "Birth intervals: structure and change." *Population Studies* 17, no. 2 (November 1963): 153–166.

SEKLANI [1], MAHMOUD, "Efficacité de la contraception: methodes et résultats." *Population* 18, no. 2 (April–June 1963). 329–348.

SHAPIRO [1], SAM, et al., "A life table of pregnancy terminations and correlates of fetal loss." *The Milbank Memorial Fund Quarterly* 40, no. 1 (January 1962): 7–45.

STIX [1], REGINE K., and FRANK W. NOTESTEIN. *Controlled Fertility: An Evaluation of Clinic Service.* Baltimore: The Williams & Wilkins Company, 1940. P. 201.

TIETZE [1], CHRISTOPHER, "Differential fecundity and effectiveness of contraception." *The Eugenic Review* 50, no. 4 (December 1959): 231–237.

VINCENT [1], PAUL. *Recherches sur la fécondité biologique. Etude d'un groupe de familles nombreuses.* Paris: Presses Universitaires de France, Travaux et Documents de l'Institut National d'Etudes Démographiques, Cahier no. 37, 1961. P. 278.

WARBURTON [1], D., and F. C. FRASER, "Spontaneous abortion risks in man." *The American Journal of Human Genetics* 16, no. 1 (January 1964): 1–25.

WHELPTON [1], PASCAL K., and CLYDE V. KISER, "Social and psychological factors affecting fertility." *The Milbank Memorial Fund Quarterly.* (Series of articles beginning in 1943 and reprinted in installments.)

WESTOFF [1], CHARLES F., et al. *Family Growth in Metropolitan America.* Princeton: Princeton University Press, 1961. P. 433.

WESTOFF [2], CHARLES F., R. G. POTTER, and P. C. SAGI. *The Third Child.* Princeton: Princeton University Press, 1963. P. 293.

Index